Learning to Get Along

Social Effectiveness Training for People with Developmental Disabilities

DONALD A. JACKSON

NANCY F. JACKSON

MARCIA L. BENNETT

DARDEN M. BYNUM

ELLEN FARYNA

Research Press   2612 North Mattis Avenue   Champaign, Illinois   61821

Cover design by Elizabeth D. Burczy
Composition by Circle Type Corp.
Printed by Malloy Lithographing, Inc.

ISBN 0-87822-326-6 (This Volume)
ISBN 0-87822-327-4 (Two-Volume Set)

Library of Congress Catalog No. 90-62603

Contents

APPENDIXES   Supplemental Training Materials

Figures

Acknowledgments

The authors wish to acknowledge two individuals for the important roles they played in the creation of this book and its companion Program Guide: David Luke, PhD, Regional Director of Northern Nevada Mental Retardation Services, for extending his interest, vision, and support to the project, and Cathy Monroe Stephens, who provided inspiration and guidance through her creative coauthorship of *Getting Along With Others: Teaching Social Effectiveness to Children* (Jackson, Jackson, & Monroe, 1983), upon which this work is based.

Numerous other individuals provided their insights and creative energy during the presentation of Social Effectiveness Training workshops and, in doing so, helped to shape this product. In particular, our appreciation is extended to Christopher McCurry, Richard Skidmore, Gary Smith, and Richard Tanner, with special thanks due to Jane Gruner for her creative help on Extended Teaching. The authors also acknowledge the invaluable contributions of many others from Sierra Developmental Center and community programs in northern Nevada.

A very special thank you also goes to our families and friends, especially Angie, Ben, Denny, Megan, Patrick, Lois, Bradley, Brenna, and Cameron, who suffered through long nights and weekends devoted to "the book." Their understanding, unending patience, and support are gratefully acknowledged.

Introduction

This book supplements the Program Guide to *Learning to Get Along: Social Effectiveness Training for People With Developmental Disabilities.*

> The Teaching Strategies and other techniques described in the Program Guide are essential to successful implementation of the group training procedures described here. If you have not yet studied the Program Guide and completed its learning activities, do so before you continue.

The format supplied here and in the Program Guide blends structured and unstructured activities so that training can occur on two levels: Individuals are taught new skills systematically and are then given ample opportunity to use them spontaneously with your guidance and support. The Program Guide provides methods for teaching social skills in the context of ongoing activities and events; this book will prepare you to use those methods for formal teaching of social skills in a small group setting.

Teaching social skills in a series of structured group sessions has two main advantages: It lets you work with a number of people at the same time, and it sets the stage for a variety of spontaneous social behaviors. This approach also brings challenges. In particular, it requires you to introduce new skills while at the same time managing and responding to ongoing behaviors. Because of the complexity of the undertaking, we recommend that you teach with a partner.

Part I of this book includes chapters to help you get your group training effort started. Chapter 1 introduces the components of a typical group training session, and chapter 2 gives step-by-step instructions for conducting a Skill Lesson. Chapter 3 highlights necessary operational preparations, both for the instructional series and for each session. Chapter 4 will guide you through a practice session before you teach a group, and chapter 5 responds to questions frequently raised about group instruction.

Part II presents session outlines based on the 21 Core Social Skills introduced in chapter 5 of the Program Guide. Specifically, each session outline does the following:

- Gives you step-by-step guidelines for conducting a Skill Lesson on a particular Core Social Skill.

- Outlines auxiliary procedures (e.g., refreshment time and activities) that reinforce the skill and create opportunities for incidental teaching to support other effective social behaviors.

- Identifies social skills that are especially important in each of these auxiliary procedures.

- Offers a context in which to teach *target behaviors*, or social skills identified as important for individual clients.

Finally, appendices provide supplementary training materials, including four scripts to teach relaxation skills, the details of activities and games used to augment the group training sessions, and a consumer satisfaction survey.

PART I
Preliminaries

CHAPTER 1

Components of the Group Training Session

This chapter describes the components of a typical group training session. We first outline a complete session to let you visualize how the components fit together, then explain in more detail how to use each of the components.

The typical group training session lasts 2 hours. Following are brief descriptions of the components and the approximate duration of each in a 2-hour session:

- *Conversation time and homework completion* (15 minutes). For participants who arrive with completed homework, this is unstructured time for talk or games. Others can use the time to practice skills and do their homework.

- *Relaxation training* (15 minutes). Relaxation techniques are taught in a progressive sequence.

- *Skill Lesson* (25 minutes). A new skill is introduced in a structured format. The lesson includes demonstration by instructors and ample role-play opportunities.

- *Refreshment time* (20 minutes). Refreshments provide an informal setting for practicing and reinforcing new skills and are a privilege contingent on participating with the group and showing competence in the new skill.

- *Activity* (25 minutes). Games, art projects, and the like provide opportunities to practice the new skill as well as skills such as compromising, sharing, and problem solving.

- *Home Notes* (15 minutes). The group completes Home Notes together to review progress toward the session's objectives and each participant's individual target behaviors. Participants share mutual approval and feedback.

- *New homework* (5 minutes). The homework for the next session is explained.

If your schedule differs from the 2-hour model reflected here, you must decide which session components to keep, how to sequence them, and whether you will use them within a single block of time or over a more extended period. To augment the Skill Lesson, you can often substitute naturally occurring events or activities for those listed in the session outline.

If you make changes in the sequence, you may wish to keep the following points in mind: First, each session component is associated with certain relevant skills in addition to the skill being taught. If you are omitting a component, plan for other opportunities to work on these additional skills. Second, in our outline, refreshment time follows the Skill Lesson. This provides a built-in way to motivate participants to work hard during the lesson. Even if your refreshment period follows an activity other than the Skill Lesson, you still may find our sequence for dismissing to refreshments a good way to structure the transition (see the section on refreshment time in Session Outline 1).

CONVERSATION TIME AND HOMEWORK COMPLETION

In the typical schedule, each training session after the first begins with a period for completing homework assigned during the previous meeting. Ask arriving participants for their homework and quickly check it for completion. Give Positive Feedback publicly to participants who have arrived with completed homework and direct them to a short reinforcing activity (e.g., a game or free conversation). This unstructured period offers the opportunity to teach cooperation, as well as showing a good attitude (Skill 1), following directions (Skill 4), joining in (Skill 10), and solving problems (Skill 14).

Participants who have not completed their homework do so with an instructor's assistance, if necessary. This homework completion segment sets the stage for teaching and practicing several skills. Because the task of completing homework is less inviting than a game or conversation, you can see how well clients follow directions (Skill 4). Inasmuch as participants are responsible for bringing the completed homework, this is a good time to acknowledge and prompt for accepting consequences with a good attitude (Skill 15) and taking responsibility rather than making excuses or blaming others (Skill 16). Finally, because some clients have difficulty remembering to complete or bring their homework, this is also an occasion to use Skill 14, solving problems, to introduce some strategies for helping them remember.

Using a Homework Progress Chart like the one illustrated in Figure 1 reinforces homework completion. Participants bringing completed homework may fill in the day's square or place a sticker on it; those who complete their homework during the free time may fill in half of the square. Each participant who completes at least 80 percent of the homework may be rewarded with a special prize at the last group session, which may include a party. The prize serves as a long-term motivator to encourage completion of the bulk of the homework assignments, whereas the free time beginning each session is a more immediate, week-to-week motivator. You may also wish to discuss selected clients' homework to reinforce their effort further.

FIGURE 1 Homework Progress Chart

21	21	21	21	21	21	21	21
20	20	20	20	20	20	20	20
19	19	19	19	19	19	19	19
18	18	18	18	18	18	18	18
17	17	17	17	17	17	17	17
16	16	16	16	16	16	16	16
15	15	15	15	15	15	15	15
14	14	14	14	14	14	14	14
13	13	13	13	13	13	13	13
12	12	12	12	12	12	12	12
11	11	11	11	11	11	11	11
10	10	10	10	10	10	10	10
9	9	9	9	9	9	9	9
8	8	8	8	8	8	8	8
7	7	7	7	7	7	7	7
6	6	6	6	6	6	6	6
5	5	5	5	5	5	5	5
4	4	4	4	4	4	4	4
3	3	3	3	3	3	3	3
2	2	2	2	2	2	2	2
1	1	1	1	1	1	1	1

Names

RELAXATION TRAINING

The relaxation training component serves a number of purposes. First, it prepares participants for the session by helping them shift gears if they have been at work or school all day. In addition, it encourages them to feel refreshed and concentrate if they are tired or keyed up. Many people—not just those with social skills deficits—become upset or angry in problem situations, and this makes it very difficult to work tcward effective solutions. Relaxation is a valuable skill that can help restore equilibrium under stress and help participants prepare for future problems by visualizing new solutions through guided imagery. The skills specifically associated with this session component include keeping hands to self, having a calm body and voice (Skill 2), following directions (Skill 4), and solving problems (Skill 14).

During the relaxation exercise, both you and the participants should be comfortable. You may have participants lie on the floor (to increase structure and minimize distractions) or sit in chairs (to make the experience more natural). Keep the room at a comfortable temperature, and perhaps dim the lights. If some participants are reluctant to close their eyes and relax, remember that people handle their feelings about relaxation in different ways. Although some people are able to relax easily, others may giggle, remain tense, feel afraid, or even fall asleep. Convey a message of understanding and acceptance by remaining calm. Speak slowly, in a soothing voice. Tell participants that it is all right if their attention wanders; just bring their attention back to the relaxation exercise.

Participants will learn to relax as they begin to feel safe and understand what is expected. You will build their confidence and understanding by using the Teaching Strategies, especially Positive Feedback. Use limited vocabulary, concrete images, and physical assistance as needed.

Appendix A provides four scripts for you to use in relaxation training. These scripts progress from introductory to more advanced techniques. The training begins with specific muscle relaxation (Script 1), progresses to deep breathing and verbal cuing (Script 2), and culminates in guided imagery (Scripts 3 and 4).

When the participants have mastered the basic relaxation techniques of Scripts 1, 2, and 3, you can tailor Script 4 to the skill being introduced in the lesson or to individual target behaviors. As written, this script refers to Skill 4, following directions. In adapting it, present problem situations and teach participants to observe their physical and emotional reactions. Then, by creating a sensory image, help them experience the situation and its resolution through use of the relevant skill. By imagining a successful experience with the skill, participants prepare themselves to have that success in reality. They experience the skill passively in a sensory, physiological, and emotional way. This relaxed practice of the skill may contribute significantly to its mastery.

You may also adapt Script 4 to help group members solve problems associated with real-life situations. For instance, if you know that Larry was recently pressured by a friend to shoplift, you can use a similar scenario during relaxation. Describe how we can tune in to our bodies to help us know when we are placing ourselves in a problem situation. Then replay the situation, showing how staying relaxed can help solve the problem—in Larry's case, by having him say no to his friend.

We encourage you to use the relaxation scripts before each Skill Lesson as well as in other situations. Depending on your expertise, you might supplement the scripts with your own ideas or with commercially available relaxation tapes. Before being too creative, however, be sure you are well informed about relaxation training methods.

SKILL LESSON

As noted earlier, structured Skill Lessons are provided for each of the 21 Core Social Skills. The purpose of the Skill Lessons is to provide an opportunity for skill learning and practice in a structured, supportive, low-stress environment. However, if the skills are to become preferred responses in naturally occurring situations that merit their use, they must be practiced frequently in progressively real situations. Part of your task is therefore to encourage this practice through incidental teaching during the training session and throughout the day.

Incidental teaching based on the Teaching Strategies is a routine part of the Skill Lesson, and a variety of skills are strengthened through its use. As a simple example, consider the following typical situation, in which two instructors are conducting a group session. One is presenting a new skill while the other is keeping an eye on the social behaviors of the group members. During a pause in the presentation, the second instructor reinforces attending behaviors by addressing the following comment to the first instructor: "_____, I noticed how David and Jennifer are showing they are listening by looking at you and staying calm." Such reinforcement opportunities are, of course, endless.

As chapter 2 illustrates, each Skill Lesson follows a standard format. The instructions to you and the suggested scripts remain the same from one lesson to the next except for what is specific to the skill being taught.

REFRESHMENT TIME

Refreshment time serves the dual function of rewarding those who have participated appropriately during the lesson and providing an excellent occasion for encouraging effective social behavior. The informality is conducive to spontaneous peer interactions; this is where the Teaching Strategies, especially the Teaching Interaction and the Ignore-Attend-Praise sequence, can be particularly useful. Valuable opportunities exist for the incidental teaching of using conversation skills, cooperating, following group rules, solving problems (Skill 14), and sharing (Skill 19).

We recommend that you make refreshment time a privilege contingent on good effort and participation during the lesson. Reward those who have done especially well by asking them to help; use descriptive praise to indicate their behavioral successes. Participants who do not initially earn refreshments may join the others by first practicing, to your satisfaction, behaviors not mastered during the lesson. Always make sure group members know they have a chance to join the others after satisfactory practice.

If group members tend to be shy and interact only with you, move away from the group until they start interacting among themselves. Float in and out as needed. With a more verbal group, join in and seize every opportunity to interrupt spontaneous interactions that are not entirely appropriate. Use Ignore-Attend-Praise to acknowledge those who are interacting appropriately and to prompt those who are not. Use the Teaching Interaction to encourage more appropriate behavior.

When refreshment time is over, ask everyone to cooperate in cleanup. Watch for those who are following directions (Skill 4) and volunteering for specific chores. Because problems frequently arise in transitions, the transition between the refreshment period and the next session component will offer even more opportunities for incidental teaching.

ACTIVITY

Planned activities provide a further opportunity to build social skills in an informal atmosphere. Appendix B describes suggested activities that prompt participants to use the skills presented in the lessons. Each activity is keyed to the skills it is designed to promote; in addition to reinforcing specific Core Social Skills, activities involve practice of such behaviors as following group rules, using conversation skills, cooperating, following directions (Skill 4), and solving problems (Skill 14).

To launch the day's activity, give the instructions and supply any necessary materials. Then join the activity and watch for opportunities to support desirable behaviors with Positive Feedback and interrupt undesirable behaviors with other appropriate Teaching Strategies. Because this part of the session is informal and fun, spontaneous peer interactions—and important teaching opportunities—abound.

Have participants clean up after activity time. The cleanup period is another transition that offers numerous incidental teaching opportunities.

HOME NOTES

Near the end of the session, bring the group back together. At this time, complete the top portion of a Home Note for each participant. (Figure 2 illustrates a completed Home Note, including comments returned by a caregiver.) Specific skills associated with this session component include following group rules, giving positive feedback (Skill 7), and accepting positive feedback (Skill 8).

Home Notes serve several important functions. When the Home Note is filled out in the group, participants receive valuable feedback and a review of their efforts for the day from other group members and from instructors. Home Notes also keep parents, group home staff, or other caregivers informed of each client's progress and alert them to the skills being taught. The reporting mechanism thus encourages group members to try the new

FIGURE 2 Sample Home Note

SKILL 4: FOLLOW DIRECTIONS

Home Note

Client Name ___Jane_____ Date __10/9/90_____

TODAY'S OBJECTIVE: Follow directions (use a pleasant face and voice; look at the person; say, "OK"; start to do what was asked right away; check back with the person when done). When you follow directions it makes you feel good about yourself; it helps you earn privileges; it keeps you out of trouble; people will like you more; people will know you are listening.

TARGET BEHAVIORS: In addition to following directions, the following individual skills were practiced.

		Score	Scale
A.	_Follow directions_	_3_	1 = completely satisfied
B.	_Ask, don't tell_	_2_	2 = satisfied
			3 = slightly satisfied
C.	_Say nice things_	_1_	4 = neither satisfied nor dissatisfied
D.	_Listen well_	_2_	5 = slightly dissatisfied
			6 = dissatisfied
E.	_Show a good attitude_	_2_	7 = completely dissatisfied

The best thing done today: ___Looked at speaker, said nice things to others._____

✂ —

PLEASE COMPLETE THIS SECTION AND RETURN

Client Name __Jane_____

SKILL 4: Follow directions

Did the participant use today's skill at least once this week?

	Yes	No
1. Use a pleasant face and voice.	✔	___
2. Look at the person.	✔	___
3. Say, "OK."	✔	___
4. Start to do what was asked right away.	✔	___
5. Check back with the person when done.	✔	___

TARGET BEHAVIORS: Use the 1–7 scale to rate the target behaviors listed above.

COMMENTS:

A. _3_   _We saw a big improvement in_
B. _1_   _following directions this week!_
C. _2_
D. _4_
E. _2_

Signature ___D. A. Jackson_____ Date __10/16/90_____

behaviors in the home setting and prompts parents and caregivers to watch for and support new behaviors. Responses of parents and others on the Home Notes provide valuable feedback to instructors. Finally, the return of the Home Note provides yet another opportunity for praise and encouragement.

You should prepare portions of the Home Note for each participant before the group meeting. Complete the demographic data and record each person's individual target behaviors from the Target Behavior Worksheet illustrated in Figure 3. (You may wish to review the discussion of target behaviors presented in chapter 5 of the Program Guide.) This will allow you and your teaching partner to focus on how each participant is progressing. If an individual seems to have mastered a skill, you may want to replace it with a more difficult one.

Home Notes can be completed more quickly if each instructor meets with half the group. Focus on one participant at a time. First ask the others to give positive feedback (Skill 7) about the person's efforts during the session; this encourages awareness of peer behavior and recognition of positive and negative behavioral components. While the feedback is being given, score the Home Note. Then ask the participant to make some true and positive self-statements. Provide some praise of your own, suggestions for improvement, and a copy of the Home Note.

NEW HOMEWORK

For every Skill Lesson, there is a homework assignment that requires participants to practice the skill away from the group and then summarize the outcome. Homework is also designed to encourage the assistance of others who will support the individual's practice of the skill in settings other than group instruction. With this assistance, the person will receive social approval and be more likely to use the new behavior in appropriate settings. Like the Home Notes component, this component is associated with the skill of following group rules.

The way in which participants do their homework will depend, of course, upon their ability to understand and communicate. Those who are capable of reading, executing the assigned tasks, and writing answers should be expected to complete the assignments independently. When those abilities are lacking, you will need to be more creative. Enlist the help of others who provide care and training. Encourage clients to ask parents, staff members, or friends for help when needed. These people can help further by arranging for additional practice of the skills included in the homework. In the process, they will become familiar with the skills being taught and be better able to support their use. If necessary, you can help with homework yourself; this will enhance communication with your client.

When you give the new homework assignment, make sure everyone understands what is expected. You may want to read the assignment aloud to the group. Anticipate the possibility that some participants may not have an occasion to try out the new skill before the next lesson: Explain that they can summarize what they would have done if they had been able to use it.

FIGURE 3   Target Behavior Worksheet

I, _____ , agree to work on improving my social skills by doing the following:
   (client name)

Target Behavior 1: _____

   which means I: _____

   (components) _____

_____

_____

Target Behavior 2: _____

   which means I: _____

   (components) _____

_____

_____

Target Behavior 3: _____

   which means I: _____

   (components) _____

_____

_____

Target Behavior 4: _____

   which means I: _____

   (components) _____

_____

_____

CHAPTER 2

The Skill Lesson

At the heart of group training is the Skill Lesson, the plan for introducing new social skills. The lessons included in this book are based on the 21 Core Social Skills; however, virtually any well-defined skill may be presented according to this plan.

The Skill Lessons use the same basic components as Planned Teaching, discussed in chapter 7 of the Program Guide, but they have a very structured format with explicit introduction and demonstration of new skills, as well as guided practice. Introducing new skills within this structure allows the client to learn in a supportive situation, thoroughly mastering the components of a new skill before attempting it during more complex interactions or under the stress of strong emotions.

The dialogue provided in each Skill Lesson is a skeleton, the *content* of the session, to be fleshed out by the *process* of the participants' ongoing behavior and the instructors' ensuing responses. Such responses should always be guided by the Teaching Strategies. Although the Skill Lesson provides important instruction, it is always secondary to the incidental teaching opportunities that occur as the participants act and react during the presentation of the lesson. It is important to avoid becoming so focused on lesson content that you lose sight of the opportunities for incidental teaching created by the communication process. Thus, the Teaching Strategies provide a method for improving clients' spontaneous social behavior as well as for managing group behavior during the lesson.

The vocabulary used in the Skill Lesson is designed to cut across age groups and functioning levels and to focus on the positive. The Skill Lesson also deals with conceptual issues: Skills are clearly defined, rationales are discussed so that participants can see the benefits of using the skill, and a dose of the "real world" is included to help prepare participants for an environment that does not always guarantee support for positive behavior.

To facilitate your learning, we have broken the Skill Lesson into five parts: (1) *skill description*, in which the skill is labeled and defined; (2) *demonstration*, in which instances of the skill (and its omission) are demonstrated and discussed; (3) *practice*, in which participants practice the skill in individualized role-play situations; (4) *rationales*, in which benefits of using the skill are stressed; and (5) *reality check*, in which potential problems are discussed.

The outline provided in Figure 4 illustrates the basic structure of the Skill Lesson. The part designations (Part 1, 2, etc.) are included in this chapter for your convenience; they do not appear in the

FIGURE 4 Skill Lesson Outline

PART 1: SKILL DESCRIPTION

Introduce skill and list components.

> Keep this discussion short and simple. Additional talk about the skill wastes valuable role-playing time.

> *Lead-in:* "Today we are going to talk about _____."

PART 2: DEMONSTRATION

Role-play appropriate example.

> With your fellow instructor, role-play the right way to use the skill.

> *Lead-in:* "This is the right way to _____."

Ask participants for skill components.

> Have the participants name the components of the skill by making positive comments about the performance. (Verbal prompting for correct answers should follow the prompting sequence described in chapter 9 of the Program Guide.) If a participant focuses on the negative (e.g., saying, "You didn't argue" or "You didn't have a whiny voice" instead of "You agreed" or "You had a pleasant voice"), use a brief Teaching Interaction to elicit more positive statements.

> *Lead-in:* "How did you know that was the right way to _____?"

Role-play inappropriate example.

> With your teaching partner, role-play the skill again, this time illustrating the wrong way to interact. This role-play highlights the differences between use and nonuse of the skill.

> *Lead-in:* "This is the wrong way to _____."

Ask participants for skill components.

> Keep this part brief, prompting as necessary. Repetition of this step is important in carrying through discrimination training and in helping to emphasize the components of the behavior.

> *Lead-in:* "What should have happened to make that the right way to _____?"

PART 3: PRACTICE

Ask participants to role-play.

Give each participant a situation to role-play. This is the most important part of the Skill Lesson; as many participants as possible should role-play at least one situation.

Lead-in: "Now it's your turn to role-play."

Ask participants to give positive feedback.

After each role-play, have participants give positive feedback (Skill 7) about the use of skill components. Group members should direct this feedback to each role-player (e.g., making eye contact and saying, "You remembered to wait for a pause" rather than looking at the instructor and saying, "He/she remembered to wait for a pause").

Lead-in: "Good role-playing. Who can tell (name role-player) what he/she did right to _____ in the role-play?"

PART 4: RATIONALES

Ask participants for rationales for using skill.

Prompt participants to describe rationales for using the skill. This helps them understand the relationship between their use of new skills and possible positive consequences.

Lead-in: "Why do you think it is important to _____?"

PART 5: REALITY CHECK

Lead participants through reality check.

With your fellow instructor, role-play a plausible interaction in which the use of a new skill does not elicit the hoped-for response. Have group members generate ideas for what to do if this happens; prompt as necessary. Remind participants that keeping calm in such a situation can help them cope.

Lead-ins: "Sometimes you might do everything right to _____, and this might happen." (Role-play scripted example.)

"You just did everything right to _____. What should you do if this happens to you?"

Skill Lessons themselves. The boldface section headings and the quoted lead-in sentences do appear in the lessons.

The quoted lead-in sentences are your basic "script." We advise that you commit the boldface section headings and these quoted lead-in sentences to memory. Memorizing the format lets you present each Skill Lesson in an automatic way and frees you for valuable incidental teaching. Many skills, including paying attention, being appropriately assertive, sitting still, and keeping hands to oneself, may be taught incidentally during the lesson if you watch for opportunities to use the Teaching Strategies.

We also suggest you role-play one or two actual Skill Lessons with your teaching partner. Take turns playing Instructor 1 and presenting the entire lesson, pausing where participant responses are indicated. Instructor 2 will have relatively little dialogue and can provide Instructor 1 with feedback. The simulated group training experience described in chapter 4 will also help orient you to the Skill Lesson format.

CHAPTER 3

Preparations for Group Training

By working through the Program Guide and the first two chapters of this book, you have oriented yourself to the components and methods involved in the group training session. This chapter will help you make necessary operational preparations before actually beginning the group. The first section discusses groundwork you need to do before the group sessions start. The second section concerns preparations for individual sessions, including selecting role-plays and supplemental activities and assigning instructor responsibilities. The final section gives suggestions for evaluating your progress in teaching social skills.

GROUNDWORK

Necessary groundwork includes recruiting and training instructors, selecting participants, deciding which skills to teach, determining each participant's target behaviors, and enlisting support from others.

Recruiting Instructors

As noted earlier, group training works better with two instructors, especially if you have clients who exhibit disruptive behaviors. If clients' problems are severe, two instructors are a must. Fortunately, the pool of potential instructors is large. It includes teachers, teachers' aides, workshop staff, students, residential or institutional staff, clinicians or therapists, social workers, parents, and others who are motivated to teach social skills. Be sure to involve coteachers in planning and preparation, both initially and as the group progresses.

Coteaching is an effective way to combine the experience of instructors. It also gives new instructors a chance to develop their skills with your support. However, the main advantage of coteaching lies in the division of labor. One person acts as lead instructor (Instructor 1), conducting the Skill Lesson and setting up the role-plays. The other serves as backup instructor (Instructor 2), providing incidental teaching, helping to present the new skill, and contributing comments and information as necessary.

The backup instructor's most important responsibility is to use the Teaching Strategies in incidental teaching. For example, by using Positive Feedback and Ignore-Attend-Praise, the backup instructor acknowledges participants who are listening, volunteering, giving on-topic answers, using eye contact, and so on. This instructor also deals with disruptive behavior or lack of attending so that the lead instructor can present the Skill Lesson as smoothly as possible. If the instructors alternate responsibilities, each can become comfortable in both roles.

It is beneficial for instructors to have prior experience working with groups. But whatever instructors' group experience, the Teaching Strategies provide the basic tools necessary for success. It is imperative that instructors complete all the activities in the Program Guide. They need this background to do effective incidental teaching, to redirect off-task behaviors, and to remain consistent, confident, and clear.

Although the group training is designed to be conducted by a team of instructors, you can present the skills alone. This simply requires giving a participant the privilege of substituting for the backup instructor in the right-way, wrong-way, and reality check role-plays. You may want to rehearse the participant's part before the Skill Lesson or simply set it up spontaneously, much like a practice role-play from the lesson. Because the lead instructor is responsible for introducing and demonstrating the skill, the participant helping you is responsible only for set-up statements.

Selecting Participants

You will need to consider many factors in making up a group. Primarily, you will want to establish a group of peers—people who will value one another's approval. You can do this by selecting individuals with shared interests and opportunities for interaction. If group members are together routinely, they are more likely to support one another's use of newly learned skills; in other words, skills practiced together in the group are more likely to generalize. Moreover, a participant who uses a new social skill outside of the structured group setting may provide a model for others who also learned the skill but lack the confidence to exercise it.

Another element of peer compatibility is age or functioning level. Generally, a homogeneous group of compatible peers simplifies teaching. Occasionally, it might be advisable to group a person with others who function at a higher or lower level. For example, some-one who is immature or intimidated by peers might be grouped with lower functioning individuals. Although this approach can ensure greater success and acceptance, you should be cautious about reinforcing immature behavior with immature models.

Whereas homogeneity with respect to peer compatibility is desirable, heterogeneity with respect to problem types is advan-tageous. A person who acts out aggressively might be grouped with others who are more withdrawn. Groups made up solely of acting-out or withdrawn individuals can yield either too many or too few teaching opportunities. Also, during a well-managed Skill Lesson, the combination of the two extremes allows modeling to occur, pulling both extremes closer to the middle. Behavioral heterogeneity also enhances response generalization as partici-pants learn to interact effectively with different kinds of people.

Optimum group size will depend on participants' functioning levels and skill deficits. If participants have relatively high cognitive abilities, you may find you can manage a group as large as 10 or 12. Lower functioning participants, who need more individual help to work on such basic skills as attending, respond better in smaller groups. Likewise, clients who present frequent behavior problems will experience more interaction in a smaller group. A ratio of six participants to two instructors will provide more frequent opportunities for role-play and practice. In addition, the smaller group allows for a good deal of incidental teaching.

Selecting Skills

The 21 Core Social Skills detailed in the Skill Lessons are arranged in a hierarchy of difficulty, with less difficult skills being prerequisite to more advanced ones. Basic skills include those essential for group participation, such as having a calm body and voice (Skill 2), listening carefully (Skill 3), and following directions (Skill 4). Participants with lower entry abilities may especially need to work on these skills before they can benefit from group instruction in more difficult skills. The Skill Lessons you choose to teach—and the order in which you choose to teach them—will therefore be based on the needs and abilities of your group.

The Core Social Skills can address many of the specific problem behaviors that your clients display. For example, those who show inappropriate expressions of anger must learn the following skills:

- Have a calm body and voice (Skill 2)

- Follow directions (Skill 4)

- Accept no as an answer (Skill 12)

- Solve problems (Skill 14)

- Accept consequences (Skill 15)

- Take responsibility (Skill 16)

- Handle name-calling and teasing (Skill 18)

- Compromise (Skill 20)

Withdrawn or nonassertive individuals must learn the following skills:

- Join in (Skill 10)

- Solve problems (Skill 14)

- Take responsibility (Skill 16)

- Say no to stay out of trouble (Skill 17)

A person entering a group living situation can benefit from these skills:

- Greet someone (Skill 5)

- Introduce yourself (Skill 6)

- Interrupt the right way (Skill 9)

- Join in (Skill 10)

- Ignore (Skill 11)

- Ask, don't tell (Skill 13)

- Take responsibility (Skill 16)

- Share (Skill 19)

- Compromise (Skill 20)

Finally, vocational success can depend on such skills as these:

- Have a calm body and voice (Skill 2)

- Listen carefully (Skill 3)

- Follow directions (Skill 4)

- Accept no as an answer (Skill 12)

- Solve problems (Skill 14)

- Ask for clear directions (Skill 21)

To supplement the Skill Lessons corresponding to the 21 Core Social Skills, you may wish to develop additional lessons to address the presenting problems and needs of your population. The list of Common Target Behaviors (see Figure 5) gives examples of other skills that can be incorporated into your curriculum. For example, clients who become upset when attention is given to others can be taught how to let others talk or let others do fun things. Those who have trouble receiving constructive criticism can be taught the skill of accepting suggestions for improvement. A quick review of this list may suggest additional skills to include.

In developing your curriculum, keep in mind the behaviors that will be supported and reinforced in the participants' everyday lives. If the skills you identify as important are not supported in the environment, additional training and coordination will be needed to ensure that such support occurs. You will need to maintain communication with others who are in daily contact with participants. You may also wish to train everyone who is involved in the participants' treatment programs (class, group home, workshop, etc.) so that a support system will evolve along with the new skills.

Select skills that will enable participants to be successful in as many situations as possible—skills that will have the most impact in everyday life. For example, a person who is aggressive may need to learn to ask, not tell (Skill 13) and take responsibility (Skill 16). However, it may be that learning to accept no as an answer (Skill 12) and accept consequences (Skill 15) will do more to alleviate the situations that usually lead to aggressive behavior. Knowing the situations that unleash problem behaviors can thus help you identify the best skills to teach.

We encourage you to rely on your creativity, expertise, and knowledge of participants in developing and sequencing a curriculum of skills. Your approach will, of course, be based on local needs. When it comes to other aspects of the program, we are much less flexible. Having seen groups fail, we are convinced that the success of your training efforts depends on following certain

FIGURE 5 Common Target Behaviors

I keep my hands to myself.	I use an inside voice.
I cooperate with others.	I use short, on-topic answers.
I volunteer.	I start a conversation and keep it going.
I take care of just myself.	I offer to help.
I join in with others.	I use positive consequences.
I let others decide.	I give suggestions for improvement.
I let others talk.	I accept suggestions for improvement.
I let others do fun things.	

Note. Skill components for each target behavior are listed in Figure 3 of the Program Guide (see chapter 5).

procedures. These include (1) using positive interactions to teach social skills; (2) carefully defining and clarifying behavioral expectations; (3) introducing new skills according to the Skill Lesson outlines to maximize experience and practice; and, above all, (4) carefully and consistently using the Teaching Strategies to ensure that participants interact positively and effectively and are supported for doing so.

Determining Target Behaviors

In choosing a curriculum of skills, you are setting priorities for the entire group. As part of your planning, you will also need to choose three to five target behaviors for each participant. These are the *positive opposite behaviors*, or behaviors deemed most important for each group member to work on. (See chapter 5 of the Program Guide to review the concept of the positive opposite.) For example, if a person has difficulty joining in conversation, a positive opposite behavior would be volunteering appropriate, on-topic responses. Briefly, target behaviors are identified through discussion with the individual and with involved professionals, parents, care providers, supervisors, and others who know the individual's skill deficits and training needs.

Take care in introducing the target behaviors. Always state them in the same way and demonstrate their behavioral components. As skills develop, you may need to revise or replace the target behaviors initially selected. If you do so, first be sure the person is using the original targeted skill consistently in everyday interactions.

Establishing Place and Time

A comfortable, natural setting will help make your training successful. Consider location, furnishings, lighting, space, temperature, access to rest rooms, and so forth. The most important requirement for your teaching setting, however, is that it be as natural as possible. A setting that reflects the conditions of your group members' daily lives will help them to generalize and use the skills they learn in the group.

Whenever possible, you should teach the group in the actual environment in which the skills will be used. For example, you might conduct sessions during a group home "family meeting," in the workshop setting, or during activity time in the classroom. You may need to get help from others in minimizing distractions such as peripheral noise and interruptions. However, the advantages of teaching where the skills will be used outweigh the inconvenience.

You will also need to give careful thought to scheduling—how long, how often, and at what time the group should meet. The complete session outline assumes a 2-hour group meeting. You can shorten that time by omitting components such as relaxation training or refreshment time, but this lessens time for incidental teaching. If you decide on shorter group sessions, be sure to compensate by building in incidental teaching during other events and activities.

The frequency of group meetings will depend on the frequency of your other contact with participants, the restrictions of your setting, the accessibility of the location to participants, and competing activities. Meeting twice a week ensures some intensity and may help improve recall and skill retention. We suggest holding weekly group meetings at minimum; longer time lapses between sessions may impede the learning process.

The optimum number of sessions depends on the participants. For lower functioning participants, you may want to limit the number of sessions to 10 or 12 and provide plenty of opportunity for skill review. Other participants may benefit from more sessions and more teaching episodes.

We suggest incorporating a review session after every four or five Skill Lessons to reinforce past learning. Review sessions also let you assess your participants' competence in using the skills you have already taught before you move on to new ones.

Getting Others Involved

Involve participants' "important others" in the program. Whom you involve and the level of their involvement will depend on your setting and the amount of time you can invest. If you work in a school setting, you will likely have access to teachers and other school personnel who interact with your participants; if you work in a large residential program, you may already have frequent contact with other staff. Involvement of others will also vary with group size. If you are teaching a small group, considerable involvement of others is possible; only limited involvement may be feasible if the group is very large.

Following are some options for eliciting the cooperation of important others.

Planning and initial assessment

The first major contribution of parents, care providers, and others is information that will help you select group participants, choose a curriculum of skills, and identify target behaviors. These people can also help as you set specific behavioral goals and decide how to measure participants' abilities, both before and after training.

Home Notes and homework

At the most basic level of involvement, others are kept informed about participants' progress in the program. Information is shared primarily through Home Notes, which briefly summarize progress and behaviors (see Figure 2). This reporting mechanism tells others what skills each participant is working on. It also alerts parents, caregivers, and others to watch for and support new skill use, informs them about the skills that are important for social adjustment, and may increase their support for the program as they acquire a sense of commitment and participation.

Before group sessions begin, meet face-to-face with parents or care providers. Describe the skills to be taught and ask the others to identify target behaviors they consider important. Explain how you will use Home Notes to share information about clients' progress in the group and to receive information about use of new skills in the natural environment. Explain the role of homework and let them know how they can help in its completion.

Follow-up contacts may also be desirable. Periodic telephone calls to parents or care providers to ask about participants' use of skills will help keep you up to date. Also periodically contact supervisors and other involved professionals to broaden the scope of two-way communication.

Planning for generalization

If possible, prepare others to reinforce the work you are doing. After new skills are introduced and role-played, ongoing incidental teaching ensures their proper use. You can use the Program Guide to train others in the application of the Teaching Strategies to provide support in the natural setting.

Adapting instruction to learners' abilities

If your clients have low cognitive functioning, limited verbal skills, or poor attending abilities, you can adapt sessions to fit their needs. We recommend a shorter session, in which you place less emphasis on verbal description and more on modeling. You can simplify skill components, homework assignments, and Home Notes. The direct involvement of caregivers will be especially important.

PREPARING FOR EACH SESSION

To prepare for each session, you will need to allocate instructor duties, select and practice role-plays, and choose activities.

Allocating Instructor Duties

If you have a teaching partner, allocate specific responsibilities before you begin the session. Assign the roles of Instructors 1 and 2, and decide who will lead other components of the session. You may also need to assign extra duties, such as bringing activity or snack supplies. Use a checklist of the jobs and assigned responsibilities to help ensure instructor readiness. The Group Preparation Worksheet (Figure 6) or a similar checklist will help you make sure that all details are covered.

Selecting and Practicing Role-Plays

Role-plays can give participants valuable practice in situations relevant both to the skill being taught and to their target behaviors. Whenever possible, the role-play situations you select should hit home. Thus, for a client who has difficulty following directions at work, you should select a role-play that represents a work situation in which that problem occurs. Each session outline includes a chart suggesting 16 possible role-play situations, grouped according to place: home, community, work, or school.

If you devise your own role-play, make it simple, specific, and short; stick to the current lesson and avoid hidden agendas that might imply additional or different skills to be learned. Initial role-plays should have a sharp focus and exclude other concerns, however legitimate they might be.

You can easily make a role-play too complex by describing a situation involving several elements. For example, this role-play for following directions (Skill 4) is unclear because it asks the client to do too many things: "Your supervisor at the workshop tells you to ask another staff person what job you should do next. That person is on the phone." To execute this role-play, the participant would need to enact both following directions (Skill 4) and interrupting the right way (Skill 9). This would undercut the purpose of the role-play—to provide an opportunity to practice the new skill in a focused, nonstressful way.

As you're selecting role-plays for your participants, think about skill limitations that may interfere with successful practice in the group. You may want to arrange seating so that participants who are likely to need extra support are placed near an instructor. Occasionally, an instructor may need to coach a role-player with a whispered verbal cue or a physical prompt—for example, gently lifting the person's chin to facilitate eye contact. (Coaching is discussed in chapter 9 of the Program Guide.) If you are working with a teaching partner, you may wish to form two smaller groups for the role-play portion of the lesson. Other suggestions for successful role-playing include placing the partners close to each other, encouraging them to use eye contact, and reminding them to maintain a serious attitude.

If your group members will have difficulty grasping role-playing because of poor communication or cognitive skills, take special care to make role-plays realistic. Have the role-players physically act out the part (e.g., come in through the door, sit at a table set for a meal, etc.). You may even need to move out of the training room to a more realistic setting.

FIGURE 6 Group Preparation Worksheet

Skill Lesson _____ Date _____

Instructions: Check off or initial to indicate assignment or completion.

_____ Instructor 1 assigned.

_____ Instructor 2 assigned.

_____ Right-way, wrong-way, and reality check role-plays selected and practiced.

_____ Participant role-plays selected.

_____ Session components assigned.

       _____ Conversation time and homework completion

       _____ Relaxation training

       _____ Refreshment time

       _____ Activity

       _____ Home Notes

       _____ New homework

_____ Home Note—copies made, names and target behaviors filled in.

_____ Homework selected and copies made.

_____ Refreshments prepared.

_____ Other _____

Choosing Activities

Specific activities to support each Skill Lesson are described in Appendix B. Select from these activities or design your own. If you design your own activities, they should reinforce the skill being taught as well as individual target behaviors. For example, if the Skill Lesson focuses on following directions (Skill 4), the activity should be one that requires participants to follow several sets of directions. Be sure to prepare before the session: Assign someone to bring necessary materials, have prizes on hand, and plan your procedures.

EVALUATION

To evaluate the effectiveness of your training, you must determine what your participants are learning and whether they are using the new skills outside of the group setting. You also need to know if they and others view the skills you teach as beneficial. Evaluations give you valuable feedback that can help you strengthen your program. They generally fall into two categories: process assessments and outcome measures.

Process Assessments

Process assessments tell you whether instruction is working so you can modify your methods as needed to enhance learning. If a participant is having difficulty mastering a skill, do you need to incorporate some Planned Teaching? Does a behavior problem identified by others suggest a particular set of role-plays that would help an individual practice and generalize a new skill? Does the group need more review to reinforce past learning? Process assessments can help give you the answers to these questions.

Such process evaluations as Home Notes and reports from teachers, parents, workshop staff, or other professionals can tell you whether participants are applying skills outside the training sessions. The Home Note gives you session-by-session information. In addition, valuable information can be gained through debriefings between instructors after each session and through frequent personal contact with those who see participants every day.

Outcome Measures

Outcome measures, conducted after the training is complete, let you know to what extent training has achieved its goals and what more needs to be done. You can find out which skills have been learned, whether they have been generalized, and whether a refresher course is needed. You can assess costs and benefits of the group training and determine the satisfaction of participants and others. In evaluating outcomes you can use a variety of methods, including interviews with participants and important others, behavior checklists and rating scales completed by those who know the participants, observation during role-play simulations, and direct observation in natural environments.

The difficulty in making outcome assessments is in obtaining useful, valid information in a practical way. Although direct observation in the natural environment might provide the best possible assessment of actual skill use, it is often impractical in clinical settings. Rating scales or simulated tests (e.g., Curran, 1982) provide a reasonable alternative.

A standardized behavior rating scale can be used if subscales cover the specific skill areas of the curriculum. Typically, a parent, care provider, teacher, or other person who knows the client well can provide the information. The Louisville Behavior Checklist (Miller, 1977) is a standardized parent report instrument useful for evaluating younger participants; it includes scales on behaviors related to our curriculum (e.g., aggression, social withdrawal, etc.). Another possibility is the Strohmer-Prout Behavior Rating Scale (Strohmer & Prout, 1989). This instrument, specifically designed to identify maladaptive behavior and personality patterns in adolescents or adults with mild mental retardation or borderline intelligence, yields a computer-generated or hand-scored report. Such rating scales can be used to screen clients for inclusion in the program; when completed both before and after training, they become a helpful means for measuring improvement.

Consumer satisfaction scales provide yet another kind of rating by people in frequent contact with participants. This type of evaluation is important because a behavioral change that you observe may have little significance if others notice no difference. Such ratings can be obtained from participants, parents, care providers, teachers, or anyone who knows the participant. The Consumer Satisfaction Survey in Appendix C rates participants on a variety of areas, such as listening, problem solving, accepting responsibility, assertiveness, and cooperation. The survey may also be used as a pre-post measure to assess skill improvement.

Records of observed problem behaviors are also useful evaluation tools if they can be maintained over a long period (e.g., in a residential institutional setting). Existing treatment programs for problem behaviors may involve the collection of data useful for your purposes as well.

These are but a few suggestions for evaluating group instruction. For further information about evaluation methods, we suggest you consult resources that treat the subject more exhaustively (e.g., Christoff & Kelly, 1983; Conger & Conger, 1982).

CHAPTER 4

A Simulated Group Training Experience

At this point, you may be wondering if you will be able to identify individual target behaviors and use the Teaching Strategies and other program methods effectively. You may also wonder how you can coordinate all these responsibilities with teaching a Skill Lesson. This chapter structures a practice opportunity to help you feel better prepared to identify and act on opportunities to teach social skills in a group setting. This practice technique may also be useful later, as a refresher.

For your practice session, we suggest that you recruit a small group of supportive colleagues, friends, family members, or others to play the roles of group participants and to observe the process. Your objective will be to present a Skill Lesson and use the Teaching Strategies to strengthen appropriate behaviors during both the structured lesson time and a more informal activity period.

In preparation for the simulated session, each of your volunteer "participants" will receive an Individual Instruction Sheet describing a client having a specific set of behavior problems (Figures 7–9). These instruction sheets, located at the end of this chapter along with other necessary materials, include a behavior-type description, appropriate target behaviors, and role-play cues. A sheet describing the "model client," a client exhibiting no particular behavioral problems, is also included (Figure 10).

> Do not look in advance at the role-play cues; your volunteers will translate them into the unanticipated behaviors that will challenge your skills during the practice session.

One of your volunteers should act as an observer, using the Observer Checksheet (Figure 11) to give you relevant feedback. This checksheet may also be used in program consultation to provide staff with continuing feedback on their use of the Teaching Strategies in the classroom, group home, workshop, or other natural site.

PREPARING FOR SIMULATED GROUP TRAINING

The following outline gives step-by-step instructions for setting up your simulated group session:

A. Recruit volunteers.

    1. Confer with your teaching partner, think of four to six volunteers who would be willing to help you for about an hour, and secure a commitment from them. Ask one to serve as observer—preferably one from whom both you and your partner would feel comfortable receiving feedback.

    2. Read over the behavior-type descriptions on the Individual Instruction Sheets. Again, *do not* read the role-play cues.

    3. Assign behavior types, using your knowledge of your volunteers. (You might regret assigning a talking-out type to a highly gregarious volunteer. Give yourself a break by selecting volunteers who will agree not to ad lib.)

B. Select a Skill Lesson.

    1. Review chapter 2, "The Skill Lesson."

    2. From Part II, select a Skill Lesson and related activity for your practice session. We suggest you use following directions (Skill 4) because it is fairly simple. Read and rehearse the Skill Lesson and activity procedures.

C. Prepare materials.

    1. Make copies of Individual Instruction Sheets. (Make extra copies of the sheet for the model client if you have more than one person playing that part.)

    2. Make a copy of the Observer Checksheet.

    3. Prepare a name badge for each participant (Figure 12).

    4. Keep this outline at hand, along with the session outline for the skill you have chosen to use.

D. Plan meeting place and time.

    1. Schedule about an hour for the session.

    2. Arrange for a carpeted room, if possible. The room should have at least 8 by 8 feet of empty space and a table with chairs for the activity.

    3. Notify your volunteers of the time and place.

E. Prepare yourself.

    1. Check your knowledge of the Skill Lesson format (see chapter 2). You should have it memorized.

    2. Study the Skill Lesson you will use in the simulated session.

       a. Memorize the components of the skill.

       b. Memorize the situations for the right-way, wrong-way, and reality check role-plays.

       c. Select role-plays for your volunteers. Use the target behaviors assigned to each to help you choose relevant role-plays. If you wish, keep the role-play chart handy or note the role-plays on index cards to jog your memory.

CONDUCTING SIMULATED GROUP TRAINING

Use this outline to help you structure the lesson itself:

A. If the volunteers are unfamiliar with the program, use the following script to open the session. If the volunteers are also being trained in the program, you may skip to the next step.

"This practice session is part of our training in the use of a program for teaching social skills to people with developmental disabilities. In our exercise today, we will be using the program format for presenting new skills. The program also specifies Teaching Strategies, which are interactions instructors use to teach and support effective social behavior as it occurs spontaneously. We will be using these strategies in our interactions with you as you act and react according to specific client behavior types. We ask that you carefully follow the instructions we will give you and avoid ad libbing. When we respond to your behavior, you should comply with our requests.

"Individuals in the program are familiar with the following group rules:

- Have a calm body.

- Follow directions.

- Look at the speaker.

- Wait for a pause.

- Stay on topic.

"In addition, they know that they will receive Positive Feedback and earn activity time by following the rules and participating in role-plays and discussions. Participants also understand that, if someone has trouble following the rules, we may use a procedure called Sit and Watch. This means removing the participant to the periphery of the group for a short time. The procedure is demonstrated to the clients during the first group session."

B. Distribute the name badges, Individual Instruction Sheets, and Observer Checksheet.

C. Review behavior types as follows:

1. Have volunteers write their own names on the name badges and put the badges on.

2. Starting with Client 1, have each volunteer read the behavior-type description at the top of the Individual Instruction Sheet. Have the volunteer illustrate the behaviors by briefly role-playing the kinds of actions typical of the client.

D. Discuss the following guidelines for volunteers:

1. Volunteers should respond appropriately at all times by looking at the speaker, sitting still, volunteering, and answering questions unless their specific instructions indicate otherwise.

2. Volunteers should respond to the instructor's prompts.

3. Volunteers should avoid stepping out of role to comment about the process or their reactions to it.

E. Have volunteers study their parts for 3 to 5 minutes.

F. Form a circle on the floor or in chairs, arranging volunteers to allow you the best use of physical prompts.

G. Teach the Skill Lesson.

H. Dismiss participants to the activity table and begin the activity.

I. Stop the session and discuss what happened. Share feedback on each volunteer's performance; especially encourage feedback to instructors. Feedback from the observer may be shared at this point or later.

FIGURE 7   Individual Instruction Sheet for Client 1

Behavior-Type Description

Client 1 is described as verbally aggressive. This person typically talks out in group and bosses other clients at work. The client's supervisor complains that the individual is belligerent and argues and pouts when corrected.

The following target behaviors have been identified for this client:

- Ask, don't tell.

- Show a good attitude.

- Follow directions.

- Wait for a pause.

Role-Play Cues

1. Blurt out, "Oh, I know, I know" for one of the first questions. Continue this each time a question is asked until the instructor praises others for quietly volunteering or says you need to have a quiet mouth. Then wait for a pause and answer questions.

2. Sigh, frown, and mumble, "You never pay attention to me" at some point when you try to get into the conversation but are ignored.

3. When you go to the activity table, tell another trainee how to do his or her job—act bossy.

FIGURE 8   Individual Instruction Sheet for Client 2

Behavior-Type Description

Client 2 has been described as withdrawn. This person typically does not volunteer at home or work, is quiet, and is almost unnoticeable in group. The client does not initiate interaction with others and tends to spend most of the time in solitary activities, such as drawing or simply staring at others. When asked a question in group or when meeting new people, the client usually blushes and answers in a soft voice.

The following target behaviors have been identified for this client:

- Speak in an audible tone of voice.
- Look at the speaker.
- Join in.

Role-Play Cues

1. Look down and do not join in unless the instructor prompts you or praises others for volunteering and looking at the speaker. If the instructor does this, gradually join in more and look at the speaker.

2. Answer in a very quiet tone of voice. Continue to do so unless the instructor prompts you to have a louder voice.

3. When you go to the activity table, sit apart from the others and do not join the conversation unless prompted to do so. (Prompts can take the form of direct instructions, instructor requests that you practice, or the offer of a reward for joining in.)

FIGURE 9 Individual Instruction Sheet for Client 3

Behavior-Type Description

Client 3 has been described as being distractible, having a short attention span, and seeming to be in constant motion. The person typically does not complete tasks and often seems to be in another world. The client appears not to be listening and gives "off the wall" answers to questions.

The following target behaviors have been identified for this client:

- Keep a calm body.

- Follow directions.

- Look at the speaker.

- Give on-topic answers.

Role-Play Cues

1. Play with your shoestrings, watch, or other article of clothing. Continue to do so throughout the lesson unless the instructor praises others for keeping a calm body or prompts you to get calm. If the instructor does this, gradually improve your sitting still. Respond to each prompt by keeping calm for longer periods of time.

2. When called on to answer a question, say, "Is it time to go yet?"

3. When answering a question (with a correct answer), look away from the person to whom you are speaking.

FIGURE 10 Individual Instruction Sheet for Model Client

Behavior-Type Description

This client exhibits very few problem behaviors. In spite of referring difficulties, the person is very anxious to please and earn activity time today, so he or she does very well on the target behaviors.

The following target behaviors have been identified for this client:

- Follow directions.
- Show a good attitude.
- Look at the speaker.

Role-Play Cues

1. Volunteer for every question asked.
2. Look at the speaker almost all of the time.
3. Keep a calm body.

FIGURE 11   Observer Checksheet

Instructions: The column at the left lists each client's target behaviors. The headings across the top list possible instructor responses. Each time an instructor responds to a client behavior, write the instructor's initials in the space below the response used and across from the appropriate target behavior. Use the "Other" column to record instructor responses to any behaviors not originally targeted. Do not record events unrelated to client behavior.

	Praises client	Praises others	Prompts	No response	Other
CLIENT 1 _____ (Volunteer's name)					
• Ask, don't tell.					
• Show a good attitude.					
• Follow directions.					
• Wait for a pause.					
CLIENT 2 _____ (Volunteer's name)					
• Speak in an audible tone of voice.					
• Look at the speaker.					
• Join in.					
CLIENT 3 _____ (Volunteer's name)					
• Keep a calm body.					
• Follow directions.					
• Look at the speaker.					
• Give on-topic answers.					
MODEL CLIENT _____ (Volunteer's name)					
• Follow directions.					
• Show a good attitude.					
• Look at the speaker.					

FIGURE 12   Name Badges for Simulated Group Experience

(Volunteer's name)

CLIENT 1

Target behaviors:

- Ask, don't tell.
- Show a good attitude.
- Follow directions.
- Wait for a pause.

(Volunteer's name)

CLIENT 2

Target behaviors:

- Speak in an audible tone of voice.
- Look at the speaker.
- Join in.

(Volunteer's name)

CLIENT 3

Target behaviors:

- Keep a calm body.
- Follow directions.
- Look at the speaker.
- Give on-topic answers.

(Volunteer's name)

MODEL CLIENT

Target behaviors:

- Follow directions.
- Show a good attitude.
- Look at the speaker.

CHAPTER 5

Answers to Common Questions

In the Program Guide and the first part of this book, we have tried to prepare you thoroughly to use our social skills program. However, we realize that you will probably have questions that we haven't anticipated. In training others, we have been asked many good questions that clarify the materials and fill in the gaps. Following are answers to some of the questions that have been raised repeatedly.

Q *What if you are working with very low functioning individuals? These techniques are fine with people who can understand and talk, but not with my clients.*

A The Teaching Strategies were developed with clients who had mild to moderate disabilities in cognitive functioning. Nevertheless, they can properly and effectively be used even with clients who have severe or profound disabilities. The principle of *shaping*, discussed in chapter 6 of the Program Guide, is especially relevant. When teaching a new skill, reinforce any approximation to the desired behavior. You can gradually raise your requirements for approval and reinforcement as the client exhibits more of the desired response.

Some of the components of the skills in the curriculum may be too complex for your clients; if so, break them into simpler components. Reduce the emphasis on verbal interaction by using physical prompts, guidance, modeling, tangible reinforcers, or any other training technique that works for the individual. Then gradually fade out the extra supports as the client becomes more proficient in the skill.

Sufficient practice is another key to learning. Clients with severe disabilities may need repeated practice in a variety of situations before they can use a new skill without assistance.

Like all training efforts with such clients, use of the Teaching Strategies must be creative, but the essential components are the same—encouraging practice of more desirable behavior and ending each interaction positively. If efforts to identify the reinforcers and teaching modalities that work with your clients do not yield immediate success, form a problem-solving group with others and discuss how the strategies can best be applied in your situation.

Q *What about group sessions? Are they appropriate for clients with lower levels of functioning?*

A Clients with lower cognitive abilities will probably not benefit from group training. The easiest way to build their social skills is through frequent and regular use of the Teaching Strategies in incidental teaching. Such teaching can be incorporated in the client's treatment plan, which specifies the individual's social behavior deficits and target behaviors. Of course, there must be consistency in the expectations of the various teachers or care providers who work with the client.

Q *What do you do about a client who has a particular problem behavior—and you've tried everything, but nothing has worked?*

A Frequently, when people complain that they have tried everything, that is just the problem. Reflect again on your use of the program. Changing behavior takes time; perhaps you have not persisted long enough with a single strategy to get results. Perhaps you are inconsistent with the client or not positive and calm in your approach, thus losing credibility. Perhaps the environment does not offer reinforcers that are interesting to the client, or your expectations for the client are unclear. If you explore these areas and still don't get results, call in an objective person to help you problem solve.

Q *What do you do if the group process disintegrates—if no one is behaving well (e.g., three participants in Sit and Watch and no one earning refreshments)?*

A Don't let this happen!

The group process may break down for many different reasons. Review the Teaching Strategies to be sure you are using them effectively. Perhaps your environment is not particularly reinforcing, or the lesson is paced too slowly, or you are emphasizing the conceptual aspects of the lesson instead of the role-playing. Maybe you have neglected to start the session with lots of recognition for positive behaviors (in particular, the readiness behaviors of looking at the speaker and having a quiet mouth and calm body).

For these or other reasons, you may find yourself with several off-task and disruptive participants. And although none may be behaving up to potential, at any given moment some will be behaving better than others. Single out those who are behaving most positively (or least negatively) and give them some special reinforcers. Let the other participants know that they too can earn these reinforcers when they have met your behavioral expectations.

Stay calm and positive. Evidence of frustration, resentment, and anger on your part will only cause the situation to deteriorate further. Your goal is not to punish, but to get the participants back on task so that they can continue to have a positive learning experience.

Q   *What if a client does not respond to Positive Feedback?*

A   Although this is not a typical problem, it does occasionally occur. We rely heavily on Positive Feedback as a reinforcer because it is easy to use, available from many sources, and a natural part of relationships.

When you use Positive Feedback to strengthen behavior, you are assuming that the person likes personal attention and acknowledgment. However, if behavior followed contingently by Positive Feedback is not strengthened, that particular form of feedback was not reinforcing. In such a case you need to observe carefully to determine what kinds of experiences the client does find desirable and reinforcing. You can then pair those experiences with Positive Feedback and gradually fade them while continuing to use Positive Feedback alone.

In addition to observing the client's response to Positive Feedback, examine your use of it. You may even ask someone to observe you. Are you sincere? Does your sincerity come across? Does your voice communicate respect for the client's efforts, or is your feedback merely a gimmick to give you control? Is there an implied judgment of the client, or are you giving feedback strictly about the behavior? Such subtle but important nuances are difficult to gain from the written page. The observations of someone whose opinion you respect will help you apply the program most effectively.

Q   *Don't clients get used to having too much Positive Feedback?*

A   We have not found this to be a problem, even though participants in our groups receive Positive Feedback from instructors about four times per minute. Praise that meets all the criteria (positive, specific, immediate, and true) provides important feedback on performance as well as indicating your pleasure; we can never get too much of this. Moreover, as we model giving and receiving Positive Feedback, our clients become more adept at the use of it. This makes them more reinforcing to be around and improves their chances for more positive social interactions in their environments.

Q   *How do you individualize role-plays for group members on the first day?*

A   If you do not know the participants and have not observed them beforehand, you will have to rely on information from other sources about their needs. In the absence of such information, choose some role-plays randomly from those included with the session outline. Soon you will learn participants' strengths and weaknesses; this will enable you to individualize future role-plays.

Q   *Should you discuss clients' feelings of anger when they are unsuccessful?*

A   Anger, frustration, defeat, or sadness expressed as a result of interactions with others yields an excellent real-life opportunity to practice constructive problem solving. Certainly a client may want to react negatively or may feel that another person deserves a negative reaction. You can acknowledge these feelings and then help the individual work out a beneficial solution. Showing empathy helps defuse the situation and refocus attention on the problem to be solved.

Q   *What do you do if the client is "antigroup"?*

A   In order to be motivated to learn and practice new skills, participants must find the group comfortable and fun—and most do. If this is not the case, try to identify the problem. The client may be embarrassed to role-play, feel out of place with the other group members, or be bored.

Some participants are unaccustomed to being in a structured environment with so many expectations, and they may be resistant and noncompliant as a result. Some may have experienced too little success and acknowledgment to become fully engaged with the group.

If you can identify the problem, you may be able to take steps to make the participant feel more positive about the group. Occasionally, however, the curriculum may not address the needs of an individual, and group training may truly not be an appropriate treatment approach.

Q   *What if a participant does not want to come to a group training session?*

A   Regular attendance ensures that participants experience continuity of curriculum and consistent work on target behaviors. It also builds familiarity among group members. When peers have formed a cohesive group, they all feel more comfortable in trying new skills.

Although some clients may voice resistance, once involved they almost always enjoy experiencing success and peer and instructor approval. Therefore, attendance at group sessions should be mandatory. The reluctant participant should be brought to the session regardless of complaints.

Most participants settle in after a few sessions. If this doesn't happen, examine other factors and consider alternate referrals. A client who persists in fighting involvement in the group is unlikely to benefit from it and may detract from the experience of other participants.

Q   *What do you do about a client who has deep-seated emotional problems?*

A   If you can see how the problems are manifested in the client's overt behavior, then you can work to remedy them. Skill deficits play an important role in emotional difficulties. Conversely, learning to interact effectively with others can help the client access reinforcing experiences; this in turn reduces the severity of the original problem.

If you suspect chronic depression or some other serious problem, it is of course advisable to refer the client to a professional with the expertise to assess and treat the problem. Group social skills training can usually occur simultaneously with individual therapy.

Q *What do you do when you have tried a particular Teaching Strategy, and it hasn't worked?*

A A Teaching Strategy will produce desired results only if you use it correctly and if it is appropriate to the situation. When a strategy does not work, you need to rethink the situation, choose a more appropriate strategy if needed, and use it in a calm, positive, and confident way. Remember to define your expectations clearly for the client, paying attention to the skills that will lead to success (e.g., listening or following instructions).

Although these strategies are designed to improve the chances that you and the client will be working toward the same end, remember that ultimately you cannot control another person's behavior. You can only control your responses and the environmental contingencies. If the client chooses another path in spite of your consistency and sincerity, recognize that the forces motivating the person are stronger than any you can offer. Let go of your need to control the client but not your consistency with rules and contingencies.

Q *Sometimes I feel sorry for a participant, and I want to bend the group rules to accommodate that person. Is this OK?*

A It is easy to get distracted by the occurrences of the moment and lose perspective. However, it is critically important to keep your long-term goals in mind and to judge situations by their future, as well as their immediate, impact. What you are asking of participants is difficult. At times the difficulty may lead to frustration, anger, and even tears and sullenness—and this may trigger your own fears about your ability to help. In such situations, determine your level of flexibility by the following criteria:

- If you feel like changing the rules because you feel sorry for the client, because you are afraid you won't be liked, or because you are just unsure of what to do, don't!

- If you feel like breaking the rules into smaller bits because you see ways for the person to be successful in smaller steps, do it!

You must be consistent with rules you believe in: Snap judgments, especially those involving all-or-nothing promises or threats, will get you into trouble.

PART II
Session Outlines

Program Introduction and Skill 1: Show a Good Attitude

> Use this outline for your first session, whichever skill you choose to teach.

PROGRAM INTRODUCTION

Introduce yourself and pass out name tags if get-acquainted segment is needed.

Instructor 1: Welcome. My name is _____ and this is _____. We're going to be meeting together (tell participants when, how often, and how many times). We will be learning some things that can help you make new friends, solve problems, and get along better with other people. Once you have learned these things, you can decide to use them with people at home and at work or school to make things go more easily for you. To help us get to know one another's names, we are going to wear name tags today.

(Pass out 3- by 5-inch cards and markers and have participants write their names on the cards, giving assistance as necessary.)

Establish rules.

Instructor 1 or 2: Before we begin today's lesson, we need to agree on some things about how the group will work. First of all, in order to make our group go smoothly, we need to have a few rules. We would like your help in deciding what rules we should have. Would anyone like to suggest a group rule?

(Call on participants attending appropriately; develop a set of rules; praise good group behaviors. Use display board or chart paper for writing rules.)

Examples of group rules:

- Have a calm body.

- Follow directions.

- Look at the speaker.

- Wait for a pause to speak.

- Stay on topic.

Define rules and ask for rationales for rules.

Instructor 1 or 2: *(Go over each rule, defining it in terms of its components; demonstrate examples of following each rule, if appropriate.)*

Why do you think it is a good idea to have these rules? *(Participants respond or are prompted.)* Following these rules is very important. When we follow the rules, everything goes smoothly, we have more fun, and we get to move on faster to other things, such as refreshments or free time. You will be earning refreshments when you follow the rules.

Introduce positive feedback.

> This step refers to Skill 7, giving positive feedback. If desired, you may model the skill at this point.

Instructor 1 or 2: When you are following the rules and trying to use a new behavior, we will let you know exactly what you are doing right. This is called *positive feedback.* For instance, right now _____, _____, and _____ are looking right at me, so I can tell they're listening. I just gave them positive feedback. Sometimes, we will ask you to give positive feedback and tell other people exactly what they did right during the lesson.

Introduce and role-play Sit and Watch.

> If necessary, review the Sit and Watch procedure described in chapter 6 of the Program Guide.

Instructor 1: Sometimes people have trouble following the rules. When this happens, the person will have to Sit and Watch. We'll show you how it works. Let's pretend that (Instructor 2) is having trouble following the rules. (Instructor 2 pokes person sitting nearby. Instructor 1 removes partner to Sit and Watch.)

Explain refreshment time.

Instructor 1 or 2: During each session we have refreshment time. The way each of you earns refreshments is by following our group rules, paying attention, practicing, and volunteering during the group. If you don't follow the rules or practice during the group, you will need to practice during refreshment time. To make sure you are able to have refreshments, what do you need to do? *(Participants respond or are prompted.)*

RELAXATION TRAINING

> In addition to today's skill and participants' individual target behaviors, give special attention to keeping hands to self, having a calm body and voice (Skill 2), following directions (Skill 4), and solving problems (Skill 14).

Instructor 1 or 2: Now we are going to do something that we will do each time we meet in the group. It is called relaxation. Relaxation teaches us how to be calm and make our bodies feel relaxed. I would like each of you to find a spot on the floor and lie down (or get your body in a relaxed position where you are sitting). Make sure that you are not touching anyone or anything. Lie (or sit) with your arms at your sides, close your eyes, and follow all the instructions. *(Have someone turn off the lights.)*

Lead relaxation training.

Instructor 1 or 2: *(Use Relaxation Training Script 1—see Appendix A.)*

SKILL LESSON

> Substitute another Skill Lesson if you are not teaching Skill 1, show a good attitude.

Introduce skill and list components.

Instructor 1: *(Ask participants to form a circle.)* Each time we meet we will learn a new skill. We will tell you about it, show you what it looks like, and have you practice it. Today we are going to talk about showing a good attitude. To show a good attitude, you:

- Use a pleasant face.
- Use a pleasant voice.
- Look at the person.

Role-play appropriate example.

Instructor 1: This is the right way to show a good attitude. I'm at work, and my supervisor is about to give me some directions.

Instructor 2: (To Instructor 1) _____, will you go over and help with those boxes, please?

Instructor 1: (Uses pleasant voice and face, looks at Instructor 1.) All right, I will.

Ask participants for skill components.

Instructor 1: How did you know that was the right way to show a good attitude? *(Participants respond or are prompted.)*

Role-play inappropriate example.

Instructor 1: This is the wrong way to show a good attitude. I'm at work, and my supervisor is about to give me some directions.

Instructor 2: (To Instructor 1) _____, will you go over and help with those boxes, please?

Instructor 1: (Makes no eye contact, does not move, whines.) All right, I will.

Ask participants for skill components.

Instructor 1: What should have happened to make that the right way to show a good attitude? *(Participants respond or are prompted.)*

Ask participants to role-play.

Instructor 1: Now it's your turn to role-play. I am going to call on someone who has been working really hard in the group today by (name specific on-task behaviors). _____ has been working really hard the whole time by (name appropriate behaviors) and looks ready to be the first one to role-play. _____, this is your role-play.

(Describe the role-play you have previously selected for this participant from the role-play chart following this session outline. Have each participant role-play the skill correctly at least once, using a previously selected situation.)

Ask participants to give positive feedback.

Instructor 1 or 2: Good role-playing. Who can tell _____ what he/she did right to show a good attitude in the role-play? *(Call on a participant who is volunteering and paying attention.)*

Ask participants for rationales for using skill.

Instructor 1: Why do you think it is important to show a good attitude? *(Participants respond or are prompted.)*

Possible responses:

- It makes you feel good about yourself.
- It helps you earn privileges.
- It keeps you out of trouble.
- People will like you more.

Lead participants through reality check.

Instructor 1: Sometimes you try really hard to show a good attitude, and this might happen. I'm at work, and my supervisor is about to give me some directions.

Instructor 2: (To Instructor 1) _____, will you go over and help with those boxes, please?

Instructor 1: (Uses pleasant face and voice, looks at Instructor 1.) All right, I will.

Instructor 2: It's about time you showed a good attitude!

Instructor 1: You just did everything right to show a good attitude. What should you do if this happens to you? *(Participants respond or are prompted.)*

Possible responses:

- Take a deep breath to get calm.
- Keep showing a good attitude.
- Feel good about what you did.

REFRESHMENT TIME

> In addition to today's skill and participants' individual target behaviors, give special attention to using conversation skills, cooperating, following group rules, solving problems (Skill 14), and sharing (Skill 19).

Decide which participants have earned refreshment time.

> Participants may earn the entire refreshment time, or they may be required to use some of this time for additional practice. Be aware of how much difficulty group members have had following rules or practicing during relaxation training and the Skill Lesson. This will suggest how much practice is needed to compensate for missed opportunities.

Dismiss participants who have already earned refreshments.

Instructor 1: OK, it's time for refreshments. (To Instructor 2) _____, who do you think has really been earning refreshments today?

Instructor 2: Well, _____ has been really following the rules, having a still body, participating, and working on (participant's target behaviors).

Instructor 1: Yes, he/she really has. And I think _____ has also done a really good job of (name specific behaviors). I'd like (first person named) to go to the table and pass out the napkins and (other person named) to go and pass out the cups.

(Continue dismissing participants to the refreshment table by giving Positive Feedback for their accomplishments and assigning each one a task. If some participants have not earned all of the refreshment time, have them practice as follows.)

Instructor 1: _____, you need to sit here with me and practice (following group rules, keeping hands to self, etc.).

(Ask questions from the Skill Lesson, have participants role-play, or lead relaxation exercises to let participants practice behaviors that were problematic during relaxation training or the Skill Lesson. Watch for good attitude and effort in practicing. Determine when each participant seems to have demonstrated acceptable competence in the skill or rule, then dismiss to refreshment time.)

Ask participants to clean up refreshment area.

Instructor 1: OK, refreshment time is over now. We need to clean up. _____, would you get the garbage can and bring it around so people can throw away their cups and napkins? *(Use the Teaching Strategies to encourage cooperation during cleanup.)*

ACTIVITY

In addition to today's skill and participants' individual target behaviors, give special attention to following group rules, using conversation skills, cooperating, following directions (Skill 4), and solving problems (Skill 14).

Suggested activities for Lesson 1: Board Games, Musical Chairs, "May I"—see Appendix B.

Explain activity for today's lesson.

Instructor 1: Today we are going to (describe activity briefly). This is a time for you to practice showing a good attitude. *(Conduct activity according to instructions given in Appendix B.)*

Ask all participants to help clean up.

Instructor 1: Now it's time for everyone to help clean up. *(Use the Teaching Strategies to help participants cooperate on cleanup. After cleanup, prompt everyone to return to the circle.)*

HOME NOTES

In addition to today's skill and participants' individual target behaviors, give special attention to following group rules, giving positive feedback (Skill 7), and accepting positive feedback (Skill 8).

Explain Home Notes.

Instructor 1: *(Hold up copy of today's Home Note.)* This is a Home Note. The last 15 minutes of the group is for Home Notes. The group members, (Instructor 2), and I will talk about how you did and give you positive feedback, and I will mark your Home Note. The bottom section of your Home Note will be marked by your (parent, group home manager, etc.), so we will know if you showed a good attitude at home. Bring this section back next time.

Divide into two groups and explain target behaviors.

Instructors 1 and 2: Every one of you has special skills that you are working on.

(Explain each participant's target behaviors, defining them in terms of their components. If two or more participants share a target behavior—for example, Skill 4, following directions—define it only once. While waiting, each participant must show patience and listen quietly. Try to mention examples of participants' use of the skills during the session, using Positive Feedback whenever possible. Encourage participants to give positive feedback (Skill 7) by describing what the person did well. Because this is the first session, score the target behaviors "n/a" for today. Inform participants about the grading scale you will use next session.)

NEW HOMEWORK

> In addition to today's skill and participants' individual target behaviors, give special attention to following group rules.

Reconvene as one group and explain homework.

Instructor 1 or 2: The homework is about today's lesson. You will need to practice at home, school, or work. Try using the new skill. Write down what happened, or get someone to help you write it down. It is your responsibility to bring your homework back completed at the beginning of our next meeting. If it is completed and returned, you will get to fill in a square on the Homework Progress Chart.

(Display Homework Progress Chart—see Figure 1. If homework is turned in late, you may want to let the participant fill in half a square.)

At the beginning of each session we will review the homework you bring back. Those who complete most of their homework by the end of all our meetings will get to choose a special prize.

Pass out homework.

Instructor 1: Here is your homework. Be sure to do it and bring it back next time. Let's see what it says. *(Read aloud and answer any questions.)* If you need help, ask your (parents, home manager, etc.).

Role-Plays

Home

At dinner, a friend talks about going to visit his family.

Your dad gives you an extra chore, but you want to go out.

Your roommate says it's your turn to unplug the toilet.

Someone else gets picked for the job you wanted.

Community

At Special Olympics practice, an athlete is showing off her medals.

While you're getting on the bus, someone accidentally bumps you, causing you to stumble.

On the way to the dentist, you forget where the office is.

The store clerk is explaining that you don't have enough money for what you wanted to buy.

Work

You wear a new dress today, and someone says she has one just like it.

Another worker is sitting in your chair at your work station.

Your supervisor tells you to work harder and not talk so much.

Your supervisor tells you to clean up the mess someone else left.

School

Your teacher is checking your homework and tells you that five answers are wrong.

People are choosing sides for a game. You are the last one chosen.

Your teacher tells you to clean up the mess you made in the sink. You want to go outside.

You are tired today and don't want to be in school. The teacher is explaining the first assignment.

Home Note

Client Name _____ Date _____

TODAY'S OBJECTIVE: Show a good attitude (use a pleasant face; use a pleasant voice; look at the person). When you show a good attitude it makes you feel good about yourself; it helps you earn privileges; it keeps you out of trouble; people will like you more.

TARGET BEHAVIORS: In addition to showing a good attitude, the following individual skills were practiced.

	Score	**Scale**
A. _____ ____		1 = completely satisfied
B. _____ ____		2 = satisfied
		3 = slightly satisfied
C. _____ ____		4 = neither satisfied nor dissatisfied
D. _____ ____		5 = slightly dissatisfied
		6 = dissatisfied
E. _____ ____		7 = completely dissatisfied

The best thing done today: _____

_____

✂ –

PLEASE COMPLETE THIS SECTION AND RETURN

Client Name _____

SKILL 1: Show a good attitude

Did the participant use today's skill at least once this week?

	Yes	No
1. Use a pleasant face.	____	____
2. Use a pleasant voice.	____	____
3. Look at the person.	____	____

TARGET BEHAVIORS: Use the 1–7 scale to rate the target behaviors listed above.

COMMENTS:

A. ____

B. ____

C. ____

D. ____

E. ____

Signature _____ Date _____

58

Homework

Client Name _____ Date _____

1. List three things you can do to show a good attitude.

   a. _____

   b. _____

   c. _____

2. Write two reasons why it is important to show a good attitude.

   a. _____

   b. _____

3. Draw a picture of a person showing a good attitude. Would you like to be with this person? Why?

General Session Outline and Skill 2: Have a Calm Body and Voice

> Use this outline for all sessions after the first.

CONVERSATION TIME AND HOMEWORK COMPLETION

> In addition to today's skill and participants' individual target behaviors, during conversation time, watch for cooperating, showing a good attitude (Skill 1), following directions (Skill 4), joining in (Skill 10), and solving problems (Skill 14). During homework completion, watch for following directions (Skill 4), solving problems (Skill 14), accepting consequences (Skill 15), and taking responsibility (Skill 16).

Conduct conversation time and homework completion.

Instructor 1: *(Collect homework and the bottom half of Home Notes from last session. Scan papers to see which participants have satisfactorily completed homework and to check Home Note comments. Ask those who have completed the homework to fill in the appropriate square on the Homework Progress Chart—see Figure 1. Direct any participants who have not completed their homework to a table, instructing them to complete the homework or practice the skill so they can join the others. Work with them as necessary.)*

Instructor 2: *(Engage participants who have arrived with completed homework in conversation, games, and so forth. This should be a fun time as well as a time to practice social skills.)*

RELAXATION TRAINING

> In addition to today's skill and participants' individual target behaviors, give special attention to keeping hands to self, having a calm body and voice (Skill 2), following directions (Skill 4), and solving problems (Skill 14).

Instructor 1 or 2: I would like each of you to find a spot on the floor and lie down (or get your body in a relaxed position where you are sitting). Make sure that you are not touching anyone or anything. Lie (or sit) with your arms at your sides, close your eyes, and follow all the instructions. *(Have someone turn off the lights.)*

Lead relaxation training.

Instructor 1 or 2: *(Use a Relaxation Training Script selected from Appendix A.)*

SKILL LESSON

> Substitute another Skill Lesson if you are not teaching Skill 2, have a calm body and voice.

Introduce skill and list components.

Instructor 1: *(Ask participants to form a circle.)* Today we are going to talk about having a calm body and voice. To have a calm body and voice, you:

- Use a pleasant face and voice.

- Take deep breaths.

- Keep quiet hands and feet.

Role-play appropriate example.

Instructor 1: This is the right way to have a calm body and voice. I'm in class, and the teacher is telling us what to work on.

Instructor 2: It's time for math, and I'm going to tell you how to do the problems.

Instructor 1: (Uses pleasant face and voice, takes a deep breath, keeps hands and feet still.) OK, _____.

Ask participants for skill components.

Instructor 1: How did you know that was the right way to have a calm body and voice? *(Participants respond or are prompted.)*

Role-play inappropriate example.

Instructor 1: This is the wrong way to have a calm body and voice. I'm in class, and the teacher is telling us what to work on.

Instructor 2: It's time for math, and I'm going to tell you how to do the problems.

Instructor 1: (Frowns, groans, moves hands and feet.)

Ask participants for skill components.

Instructor 1: What should have happened to make that the right way to have a calm body and voice? *(Participants respond or are prompted.)*

Ask participants to role-play.

Instructor 1: Now it's your turn to role-play. I am going to call on someone who has been working really hard in the group today by (name specific on-task behaviors). _____ has been working really hard the whole time by (name appropriate behaviors) and looks ready to be the first one to role-play. _____, this is your role-play.

(Describe the role-play you have previously selected for this participant from the role-play chart following this session outline. Have each participant role-play the skill correctly at least once, using a previously selected situation.)

Ask participants to give positive feedback.

Instructor 1 or 2: Good role-playing. Who can tell _____ what he/she did right to have a calm body and voice in the role-play? *(Call on a participant who is volunteering and paying attention.)*

Ask participants for rationales for using skill.

Instructor 1: Why do you think it is important to have a calm body and voice? *(Participants respond or are prompted.)*

Possible responses:

- It makes you feel good about yourself.

- It helps you earn privileges.

- It keeps you out of trouble.

- People will know you are listening.

Lead participants through reality check.

Instructor 1: Sometimes you try really hard to have a calm body and voice, and this might happen. I'm in class, and the teacher is telling us what to work on.

Instructor 2: It's time for math, and I'm going to tell you how to do the problems.

Instructor 1: (Uses pleasant face and voice, takes a deep breath, keeps hands and feet still.) OK, _____.

Instructor 2: _____, you need to be listening to me so you don't make mistakes!

Instructor 1: You just did everything right to have a calm body and voice. What should you do if this happens to you? *(Participants respond or are prompted.)*

Possible responses:

- Take a deep breath to get calm.

- Show a good attitude.

- Feel good about what you did.

- Keep trying to have a calm body and voice.

REFRESHMENT TIME

> In addition to today's skill and participants' individual target behaviors, give special attention to using conversation skills, cooperating, following group rules, solving problems (Skill 14), and sharing (Skill 19).

Decide which participants have earned refreshment time.

> Participants may earn the entire refreshment time, or they may be required to use some of this time for additional practice. Be aware of how much difficulty group members have had following rules or practicing during relaxation training and the Skill Lesson. This will suggest how much practice is needed to compensate for missed opportunities.

Dismiss participants who have already earned refreshments.

Instructor 1: OK, it's time for refreshments. (To Instructor 2) _____, who do you think has really been earning refreshments today?

Instructor 2: Well, _____ has been really following the rules, having a still body, participating, and working on (participant's target behaviors).

Instructor 1: Yes, he/she really has. And I think _____ has also done a really good job of (name specific behaviors). I'd like (first person named) to go to the table and pass out the napkins and (other person named) to go and pass out the cups.

(Continue dismissing participants to the refreshment table by giving them Positive Feedback for their accomplishments and assigning each one a task. If some participants have not earned all of the refreshment time, have them practice as follows.)

Instructor 1: _____, you need to sit here with me and practice (following group rules, keeping hands to self, etc.).

(Ask questions from the Skill Lesson, have participants role-play, or lead relaxation exercises to let participants practice behaviors that were problematic during relaxation training or the Skill Lesson. Watch for good attitude and effort in practicing. Determine when each participant seems to have demonstrated acceptable competence in the skill or rule, then dismiss to refreshment time.)

Ask participants to clean up refreshment area.

Instructor 1: OK, refreshment time is over now. We need to clean up. _____, would you get the garbage can and bring it around so people can throw away their cups and napkins? *(Use the Teaching Strategies to encourage cooperation during cleanup.)*

ACTIVITY

> In addition to today's skill and participants' individual target behaviors, give special attention to following group rules, using conversation skills, cooperating, following directions (Skill 4), and solving problems (Skill 14).
>
> Suggested activities for Lesson 2: Board Games, Spoons—see Appendix B.

Explain activity for today's lesson.

Instructor 1: Today we are going to (describe activity briefly). This is a time for you to practice having a calm body and voice. *(Conduct activity according to instructions given in Appendix B).*

Ask all participants to help clean up.

Instructor 1: Now it's time for everyone to help clean up. *(Use the Teaching Strategies to help participants cooperate on cleanup. After cleanup, prompt everyone to return to the circle.)*

HOME NOTES

In addition to today's skill and participants' individual target behaviors, give special attention to following group rules, giving positive feedback (Skill 7), and accepting positive feedback (Skill 8).

Divide into two groups and score Home Notes.

Instructors 1 and 2: _____, we are going to talk about how you did during today's session. Who can give _____ some positive feedback and tell some good things about how he/she did on (the target behaviors)?

(Score the top half of the Home Note while the others are giving positive feedback. Ask for specific feedback for each of the participant's target behaviors and add your own comments, pointing out progress and areas needing improvement.)

(To the same participant) _____, now what do you think was the best thing you did in group today? *(Participant responds or is prompted.)*

Instructors 1 and 2: That's good. *(Add specific descriptions of strong points.)* You might also try to (give participant suggestions for improvement). Here is your Home Note. *(Repeat sequence with each participant.)*

NEW HOMEWORK

In addition to today's skill and participants' individual target behaviors, give special attention to following group rules.

Reconvene as one group and pass out homework.

Instructor 1: Here is your homework. Be sure to do it and bring it back next time. Let's see what it says. *(Read aloud and answer any questions.)* If you need help, ask your (parents, teacher, home manager, etc.).

Role-Plays

Home

Your roommate accidentally drops and breaks your favorite cup.

You are watching TV, and your roommate changes the channel.

You're cooking your dinner and watching TV, and your dinner burns.

The toilet overflows, and you're embarrassed.

Community

You're at a restaurant. The waitress is really nice, but she gets your order wrong.

You are bowling, and your last time up everyone laughed at you for doing poorly.

You're in line at the movie, and the guy in front of you lets six friends in line ahead of you.

You are at the checkstand ready to pay for your basket full of groceries, but you're $2.00 short.

Work

Your boss gives you some instructions about your work, but when you try to do it, you realize you didn't understand.

You run out of parts before you finish a job, and you're in a hurry to leave.

You stopped to talk to friends on the way back from your break. Your boss says you will lose some time from your lunch hour.

Your supervisor says either you or your coworker can go on a break when you finish a project. Your coworker finishes first.

School

You turn in your assignment, and your teacher says you did the wrong page.

Your teacher says the first one done with the math page gets to help set up the movie. Your friend finishes first.

You forgot your point sheet, and your teacher asks where it is.

You a have a substitute teacher who doesn't understand that it's your turn to help at lunch, and she picks someone else.

SKILL 2: HAVE A CALM BODY AND VOICE **Home Note**

Client Name _____ Date _____

TODAY'S OBJECTIVE: Have a calm body and voice (use a pleasant face and voice; take deep breaths; keep quiet hands and feet). When you have a calm body and voice it makes you feel good about yourself; it helps you earn privileges; it keeps you out of trouble; people will know you are listening.

TARGET BEHAVIORS: In addition to having a calm body and voice, the following individual skills were practiced.

	Score	**Scale**
A. _____ ____	1 = completely satisfied
B. _____ ____	2 = satisfied
	3 = slightly satisfied
C. _____ ____	4 = neither satisfied nor dissatisfied
D. _____ ____	5 = slightly dissatisfied
	6 = dissatisfied
E. _____ ____	7 = completely dissatisfied

The best thing done today: _____

_____

✂ —

PLEASE COMPLETE THIS SECTION AND RETURN

Client Name _____

SKILL 2: Have a calm body and voice

Did the participant use today's skill at least once this week?

	Yes	No
1. Use a pleasant face and voice.	____	____
2. Take deep breaths.	____	____
3. Keep quiet hands and feet.	____	____

TARGET BEHAVIORS: Use the 1–7 scale to rate the target behaviors listed above.

COMMENTS:

A. ____

B. ____

C. ____

D. ____

E. ____

Signature _____ Date _____

SKILL 2: HAVE A CALM BODY AND VOICE

Homework

Client Name _____ Date _____

1. Sometime this week, practice taking deep breaths. How did breathing make you feel?

_____

_____

_____

_____

_____

_____

2. Write down two times when you need to have a calm body and voice.

   a. _____

   b. _____

3. Why is it a good idea to have a calm body and voice, even if you are upset?

_____

_____

_____

_____

_____

Skill 3: Listen Carefully

> Follow the instructions provided in Session Outline 2 for conducting • Conversation Time and Homework Completion and • Relaxation Training. Then go on to the • Skill Lesson.

SKILL LESSON

Introduce skill and list components.

Instructor 1: *(Ask participants to form a circle.)* Today we are going to talk about listening carefully. To listen carefully, you:

- Use a pleasant face.

- Look at the person.

- Keep a quiet mouth.

- Keep quiet hands and body.

Role-play appropriate example.

Instructor 1: This is the right way to listen carefully. My supervisor is explaining how to do a new job.

Instructor 2: OK, you need to strip the insulation off the blue and green wires, starting one inch from the end of the wire.

Instructor 1: (Uses pleasant face, looks at Instructor 2, and keeps a quiet mouth, hands, and body.)

Ask participants for skill components.

Instructor 1: How did you know that was the right way to listen carefully? *(Participants respond or are prompted.)*

Role-play inappropriate example.

Instructor 1: This is the wrong way to listen carefully. My supervisor is explaining how to do a new job.

Instructor 2: OK, you need to strip the insulation off the blue and green wires, starting one inch from the end of the wire.

Instructor 1: (Looks away, grimaces, fidgets.) I don't want to.

Ask participants for skill components.

> Instructor 1: What should have happened to make that the right way to listen carefully? *(Participants respond or are prompted.)*

Ask participants to role-play.

> Instructor 1: Now it's your turn to role-play. I am going to call on someone who has been working really hard in the group today by (name specific on-task behaviors). _____ has been working really hard the whole time by (name appropriate behaviors) and looks ready to be the first one to role-play. _____, this is your role-play.
>
> *(Describe the role-play you have previously selected for this participant from the role-play chart following this session outline. Have each participant role-play the skill correctly at least once, using a previously selected situation.)*

Ask participants to give positive feedback.

> Instructor 1 or 2: Good role-playing. Who can tell _____ what he/she did right to listen carefully in the role-play? *(Call on a participant who is volunteering and paying attention.)*

Ask participants for rationales for using skill.

> Instructor 1: Why do you think it is important to listen carefully? *(Participants respond or are prompted.)*
>
> Possible responses:
>
> - You won't make mistakes as often.
> - People will know you heard them.
> - You will know what people want you to do.
> - People will like you.

Lead participants through reality check.

> Instructor 1: Sometimes you try really hard to listen carefully, and this might happen. My supervisor is explaining how to do a new job.
>
> Instructor 2: OK, you need to strip the insulation off the blue and green wires, starting one inch from the end of the wire.
>
> Instructor 1: (Uses pleasant face, looks at Instructor 2, and keeps a quiet mouth, hands, and body.)
>
> Instructor 2: Now, _____, I hope you can get it right this time!
>
> Instructor 1: You just did everything right to listen carefully. What should you do if this happens to you? *(Participants respond or are prompted.)*

Possible responses:

- Take a deep breath to get calm.

- Show a good attitude.

- Feel good about what you did.

- Keep listening carefully.

- Say, "I will!"

Follow the instructions provided in Session Outline 2 for conducting • Refreshment Time • Activity • Home Notes and • New Homework.

Suggested activities for Session 3: Simon Says, Telephone—see Appendix B.

Role-Plays

Home

Your home manager wants you to clean the refrigerator. You have never done that before. He/she tells you what to do.

Your roommate is explaining to you how he/she wants to divide up the closet space.

During a family meeting, others are offering ideas on what movie to see together this weekend.

Your parents are going out for the evening. Your dad is explaining what you can have for dinner.

Community

You ask a store clerk, "Where is the laundry soap?" He/she tells you it is in aisle 12A on the second shelf.

You got on the wrong bus, so you ask the bus driver how to get back to the transfer stop.

You just moved into a group home and don't know where the grocery store is. Your roommate tells you.

You are out to dinner with friends. You ask the waitress where the rest rooms are.

Work

Your supervisor is talking to your work group about safety around the shrink-wrap machine.

Your supervisor is describing a task on a new machine for you.

Your job coach is telling you a new way to pack boxes. You already know one way to do it.

A coworker is telling you what a good job you are doing: thorough, steady, with no mistakes . . .

School

Your teacher is giving a list of things to bring for tomorrow's class trip: bag lunch, jacket, $2.00 admission to the planetarium . . .

The coach is giving new rules for playing basketball: no dribbling this game.

The principal is making morning announcements over the loudspeaker in homeroom.

The bell rings for a fire drill. Your teacher is giving directions to a different exit.

SKILL 3: LISTEN CAREFULLY   # Home Note

Client Name _____ Date _____

TODAY'S OBJECTIVE: Listen carefully (use a pleasant face; look at the person; keep a quiet mouth; keep quiet hands and body). When you listen carefully you won't make mistakes as often; people will know you heard them; you will know what people want you to do; people will like you.

TARGET BEHAVIORS: In addition to listening carefully, the following individual skills were practiced.

		Score	**Scale**
A.	_____	____	1 = completely satisfied
B.	_____	____	2 = satisfied
			3 = slightly satisfied
C.	_____	____	4 = neither satisfied nor dissatisfied
D.	_____	____	5 = slightly dissatisfied
			6 = dissatisfied
E.	_____	____	7 = completely dissatisfied

The best thing done today: _____

_____

✂ –

PLEASE COMPLETE THIS SECTION AND RETURN

Client Name _____

SKILL 3: Listen carefully

Did the participant use today's skill at least once this week?

	Yes	No
1. Use a pleasant face and voice.	____	____
2. Look at the person.	____	____
3. Keep a quiet mouth.	____	____
4. Keep quiet hands and body.	____	____

TARGET BEHAVIORS: Use the 1–7 scale to rate the target behaviors listed above.

COMMENTS:

A. ____

B. ____

C. ____

D. ____

E. ____

Signature _____ Date _____

Homework

Client Name _____ Date _____

1. Tell about two times when you listened carefully this week.

   Time 1:

   a. Where were you?_____

   b. What did you do to listen carefully?_____

   _____

   _____

   _____

   Time 2:

   a. Where were you?_____

   b. What did you do to listen carefully?_____

   _____

   _____

   _____

2. Why is it important to listen carefully?

   _____

   _____

   _____

   _____

   _____

Skill 4: Follow Directions

> Follow the instructions provided in Session Outline 2 for conducting • Conversation Time and Homework Completion and • Relaxation Training. Then go on to the • Skill Lesson.

SKILL LESSON

Introduce skill and list components.

Instructor 1: *(Ask participants to form a circle.)* Today we are going to talk about how to follow directions. To follow directions, you:

- Use a pleasant face and voice.

- Look at the person.

- Say, "OK."

- Start to do what was asked right away.

- Check back with the person when done.

Role-play appropriate example.

Instructor 1: This is the right way to follow directions. I'm at work, and my supervisor is about to give me some directions.

Instructor 2: (To Instructor 1) _____, break is over and you need to go back to work now.

Instructor 1: OK. (Gets up right away, goes to work, then raises hand.) I'm ready to work now.

Ask participants for skill components.

Instructor 1: How did you know that was the right way to follow directions? *(Participants respond or are prompted.)*

Role-play inappropriate example.

Instructor 1: This is the wrong way to follow directions. I'm at work, and my supervisor is about to give me some directions.

Instructor 2: (To Instructor 1) _____, break is over and you need to go back to work now.

Instructor 1: OK. (No eye contact, does not move, continues to do what he/she was doing.)

Ask participants for skill components.

Instructor 1: What should have happened to make that the right way to follow directions? *(Participants respond or are prompted.)*

Ask participants to role-play.

Instructor 1: Now it's your turn to role-play. I am going to call on someone who has been working really hard in the group today by (name specific on-task behaviors). _____ has been (name appropriate behaviors) and looks ready to be the first one to role-play. _____, this is your role-play.

(Describe the role-play you have previously selected for this participant from the role-play chart following this session outline. Have each participant role-play the skill correctly at least once, using a previously selected situation.)

Ask participants to give positive feedback.

Instructor 1 or 2: Good role-playing. Who can tell _____ what he/she did right to follow directions in the role-play? *(Call on a participant who is volunteering and paying attention.)*

Ask participants for rationales for using skill.

Instructor 1: Why do you think it is important to follow directions? *(Participants respond or are prompted.)*

Possible responses:

- It makes you feel good about yourself.

- It helps you earn privileges.

- It keeps you out of trouble.

- People will like you more.

- People will know you are listening.

Lead participants through reality check.

Instructor 1: Sometimes you try really hard to follow directions, and this might happen. I'm at work, and my supervisor is about to give me some directions.

Instructor 2: (To Instructor 1) _____, break is over and you need to go back to work now.

Instructor 1: OK. (Gets up right away, goes back to work, then raises hand.) I'm ready to work now.

Instructor 2: It's about time you followed my directions!

Instructor 1: You just did everything right to follow directions. What should you do if this happens to you? *(Participants respond or are prompted.)*

Possible responses:

- Take a deep breath to get calm.

- Show a good attitude.

- Feel good about what you did.

- Keep trying to follow directions.

Follow the instructions provided in Session Outline 2 for conducting • Refreshment Time • Activity • Home Notes and • New Homework.

Suggested activities for Session 4: Simon Says, Directed Drawing, Marble Game—see Appendix B.

Role-Plays

Home

Your father tells you to clean up your room before you go out with your friend. Your friend is waiting for you.

Your resident manager asks you to introduce your new friend and invite him to dinner.

Your mother tells you to boil the eggs for tuna salad.

Your home supervisor compliments you on how your hair looks and then tells you to shave again.

Community

A friend hands you his new magazine and tells you to give it back as soon as you've looked at it.

The park supervisor asks you to help others clean up after the picnic.

The ticket seller tells you to go to the end of the line.

Your group home manager asked you to call if you will be home late. You missed the bus and have to wait for the next one.

Work

Your supervisor tells you to find another person and unload some heavy boxes. You've worked hard already, and you're tired.

Your boss tells you to finish the work in the back room before you come out and join the others in the lunch room.

Yesterday you had an argument with your coworker. Today your supervisor asks you to apologize.

Your supervisor asks you to help a coworker clean the lunch room.

School

The captain of the team you are on tells you to wait your turn and not try to get ahead in line.

Your teacher tells the whole class to clean up after art. You didn't make the mess.

Your teacher tells you to clean up the mess you made in the sink.

Your teacher tells you to choose a partner and lead a game in front of the class.

Home Note

Client Name _____ Date _____

TODAY'S OBJECTIVE: Follow directions (use a pleasant face and voice; look at the person; say, "OK"; start to do what was asked right away; check back with the person when done). When you follow directions it makes you feel good about yourself; it helps you earn privileges; it keeps you out of trouble; people will like you more; people will know you are listening.

TARGET BEHAVIORS: In addition to following directions, the following individual skills were practiced.

	Score	Scale
A. _____	____	1 = completely satisfied
B. _____	____	2 = satisfied
		3 = slightly satisfied
C. _____	____	4 = neither satisfied nor dissatisfied
D. _____	____	5 = slightly dissatisfied
		6 = dissatisfied
E. _____	____	7 = completely dissatisfied

The best thing done today: _____

_____

✂ —

PLEASE COMPLETE THIS SECTION AND RETURN

Client Name _____

SKILL 4: Follow directions

Did the participant use today's skill at least once this week?

	Yes	No
1. Use a pleasant face and voice.	____	____
2. Look at the person.	____	____
3. Say, "OK."	____	____
4. Start to do what was asked right away.	____	____
5. Check back with the person when done.	____	____

TARGET BEHAVIORS: Use the 1–7 scale to rate the target behaviors listed above.

COMMENTS:

A. ____
B. ____
C. ____
D. ____
E. ____

Signature _____ Date _____

81

Homework

Client Name _____ Date _____

1. What are five things you can do to show that you are following directions the right way?

   a. _____

   b. _____

   c. _____

   d. _____

   e. _____

2. Write down a direction someone at home gave to you. What exactly did the person say? What did you say and do?

   _____

   _____

   _____

   _____

3. Write down a direction your supervisor at work or some other person gave you. What exactly did the person say? What did you say and do?

   _____

   _____

   _____

   _____

4. What should you do and/or say if someone gives you a direction but you don't want to do it? (Tell why you answered this way.)

   _____

   _____

   _____

   _____

Skill 5: Greet Someone

> Follow the instructions provided in Session Outline 2 for conducting • Conversation Time and Homework Completion and • Relaxation Training. Then go on to the • Skill Lesson.

SKILL LESSON

Introduce skill and list components.

Instructor 1: *(Ask participants to form a circle.)* Today we are going to talk about how to greet someone you already know. To greet someone, you:

- Use a pleasant face and voice.
- Keep a calm body.
- Look at the person.
- Greet the person by saying something like "Hi, how are you?"

Role-play appropriate example.

Instructor 1: This is the right way to greet someone. I'm at my work station and my coworker, (Instructor 2), is coming in. (Looks at Instructor 2, uses pleasant face and voice.) Hi, how are you this morning?

Ask participants for skill components.

Instructor 1: How did you know that was the right way to greet someone? *(Participants respond or are prompted.)*

Role-play inappropriate example.

Instructor 1: This is the wrong way to greet someone. I'm at my work station and my coworker, (Instructor 2), is coming in. (Looks at Instructor 2, frowns, uses a loud voice.) Where have you been? I've been looking for you!

Ask participants for skill components.

Instructor 1: What should have happened to make that the right way to greet someone? *(Participants respond or are prompted.)*

Ask participants to role-play.

Instructor 1: Now it's your turn to role-play. I am going to call on someone who has been working really hard in the group today by (name specific on-task behaviors). _____ has been (name appropriate behaviors) and looks ready to be the first one to role-play. _____, this is your role-play.

(Describe the role-play you have previously selected for this participant from the role-play chart following this session outline. Have each participant role-play the skill correctly at least once, using a previously selected situation.)

Ask participants to give positive feedback.

Instructor 1 or 2: Good role-playing. Who can tell _____ what he/she did right to greet someone in the role-play? *(Call on a participant who is volunteering and paying attention.)*

Ask participants for rationales for using skill.

Instructor 1: Why do you think it is important to greet someone? *(Participants respond or are prompted.)*

Possible responses:

- You will seem friendlier.

- People will like to talk to you.

- You will have more friends.

- People will like you because you are polite.

Lead participants through reality check.

Instructor 1: Sometimes you try really hard to greet someone, and this might happen. I'm at my work station, and my coworker, (Instructor 2), is coming in. (Looks at Instructor 2, uses pleasant face and voice.) Hi, how are you this morning?

Instructor 2: Leave me alone. Get lost!

Instructor 1: You just did everything right to greet someone. What should you do if this happens to you? *(Participants respond or are prompted.)*

Possible responses:

- Take a deep breath to get calm.

- Show a good attitude.

- Feel good about being polite.

- Ignore.

- Go find a friendlier person.

Follow the instructions provided in Session Outline 2 for conducting • Refreshment Time • Activity • Home Notes and • New Homework.

Suggested activity for Session 5: Greeting Game—see Appendix B.

Role-Plays

Home

Your father arrives home from work. You are watching TV.

When your roommate answers the doorbell, it's a friend of hers you've met before. You're in the next room.

A relative you haven't seen for a while comes to your house. He is talking to someone.

You're in the yard. A person you know from work comes by on her bike.

Community

As you get on the bus you always ride, your regular bus driver smiles at you.

You're at the regional center waiting for an appointment; you know lots of people. Someone you know walks by.

At the park, a person you know from a class you took walks by.

You're at the supermarket, and you recognize a neighbor.

Work

When you walk into work in the morning, your supervisor is standing there.

After you sit down at your work station, your coworkers come in and join you.

While you're at work, a social worker you know comes by your work station.

A friend you haven't seen today sits by you at lunch.

School

Your teacher is writing on the chalkboard as you enter the classroom in the morning.

At recess, you see a friend from another class.

A teacher from another class comes in. She is talking to your teacher.

You're walking down the hall. A person you would like to know is coming toward you.

Home Note

Client Name _____ Date _____

TODAY'S OBJECTIVE: Greet someone (use a pleasant face and voice; keep a calm body; look at the person; greet the person by saying something like "Hi, how are you?"). When you greet people you will seem friendlier; people will like to talk to you; you will have more friends; people will like you because you are polite.

TARGET BEHAVIORS: In addition to greeting someone, the following individual skills were practiced.

	Score	**Scale**
A. _____	_____	1 = completely satisfied
B. _____	_____	2 = satisfied
		3 = slightly satisfied
C. _____	_____	4 = neither satisfied nor dissatisfied
D. _____	_____	5 = slightly dissatisfied
		6 = dissatisfied
E. _____	_____	7 = completely dissatisfied

The best thing done today: _____

_____

✂ –

PLEASE COMPLETE THIS SECTION AND RETURN

Client Name _____

SKILL 5: Greet someone

Did the participant use today's skill at least once this week?

	Yes	No
1. Use a pleasant face and voice.	____	____
2. Keep a calm body.	____	____
3. Look at the person.	____	____
4. Greet the person by saying something like "Hi, how are you?"	____	____

TARGET BEHAVIORS: Use the 1–7 scale to rate the target behaviors listed above.

COMMENTS:

A. _____

B. _____

C. _____

D. _____

E. _____

Signature _____ Date _____

SKILL 5: GREET SOMEONE   # Homework

Client Name _____ Date _____

1. What are two ways you can greet someone you know?

   a. _____

   b. _____

2. Why is it important to greet people when you first see them? What might happen if you begin talking without greeting someone first?

   _____

   _____

   _____

   _____

   _____

3. Practice greeting someone you know the right way.

   a. Whom did you greet? _____

   b. What did you say and do? _____

   _____

   _____

   _____

   c. What did the other person say and do? _____

   _____

   _____

   _____

Skill 6: Introduce Yourself

> Follow the instructions provided in Session Outline 2 for conducting • Conversation Time and Homework Completion and • Relaxation Training. Then go on to the • Skill Lesson.

SKILL LESSON

Introduce skill and list components.

Instructor 1: *(Ask participants to form a circle.)* Today we are going to talk about how to introduce yourself. To introduce yourself, you:

- Use a pleasant face and voice.
- Look at the person.
- Tell the person your name.
- Ask for the person's name.

Role-play appropriate example.

Instructor 1: This is the right way to introduce yourself. I'm going to introduce myself to a new student. (To Instructor 2) Hi, my name is ———————. What's yours?

Instructor 2: I'm ———————. Nice to meet you.

Ask participants for skill components.

Instructor 1: How did you know that was the right way to introduce yourself? *(Participants respond or are prompted.)*

Role-play inappropriate example.

Instructor 1: This is the wrong way to introduce yourself. I'm going to introduce myself to a new student. (To Instructor 2) Hey, are you new here?

Instructor 2: Yeah.

Ask participants for skill components.

Instructor 1: What should have happened to make that the right way to introduce yourself? *(Participants respond or are prompted.)*

Ask participants to role-play.

Instructor 1: Now it's your turn to role-play. I am going to call on someone who has been working really hard in the group today by (name specific on-task behaviors). _____ has been (name appropriate behaviors) and looks ready to be the first one to role-play. _____, this is your role-play.

(Describe the role-play you have previously selected for this participant from the role-play chart following this session outline. Have each participant role-play the skill correctly at least once, using a previously selected situation.)

Ask participants to give positive feedback.

Instructor 1 or 2: Good role-playing. Who can tell _____ what he/she did right to introduce himself/herself in the role-play? *(Call on a participant who is volunteering and paying attention.)*

Ask participants for rationales for using skill.

Instructor 1: Why do you think it is important to introduce yourself the right way? *(Participants respond or are prompted.)*

Possible responses:

- You will know the person's name.

- You will seem friendlier.

- You will have more friends.

- People will like you because you are polite.

Lead participants through reality check.

Instructor 1: Sometimes you try really hard to introduce yourself, and this might happen. I'm going to introduce myself to a new student. (To Instructor 2) Hi, my name is _____. What's yours?

Instructor 2: Oh, leave me alone. Get lost!

Instructor 1: You just did everything right to introduce yourself. What should you do if this happens to you? *(Participants respond or are prompted.)*

Possible responses:

- Take a deep breath to get calm.

- Show a good attitude.

- Ignore.

- Find a friendlier person.

- Wait until a better time.

Follow the instructions provided in Session Outline 2 for conducting • Refreshment Time • Activity • Home Notes and • New Homework.

Suggested activity for Session 6: Name Game—see Appendix B.

Role-Plays

Home

Your sister has a new friend over. They are having a snack, and you'd like to join them.

You go to a meeting at another apartment. You see a person there you haven't met.

You're at the group home. Another resident's mother comes in. You haven't met her.

You and your roommate are having a party. You haven't met some of your roommate's friends.

Community

You see the same person each day at the bus stop. You'd like to get to know him.

You are at the beach. Some people near you ask if you'd like to join them.

You are playing video games at the arcade. You see someone you have often seen before.

At the grocery store you are standing in line behind someone you met at work last week. You've forgotten her name.

Work

There are two new employees at the workshop today. You see one of them sitting alone in the lunch room.

You're working a different shift today. You want to get to know one of the other employees.

At work, you're talking to a friend. A new person walks up and wants to know how to get to the cafeteria.

There is a new supervisor at work. You need to ask a question about the project you're working on.

School

Your teacher sends you into another classroom to help out with younger students. You haven't met the teacher.

You need some help with the reading assignment. There is a new student aide whom you haven't met.

Your teacher assigns everyone in the class to work in small groups. You only know one of the people in your group.

You see a new student on the playground. You have a basketball and would like to shoot some baskets.

SKILL 6: INTRODUCE YOURSELF   # Home Note

Client Name _____ Date _____

TODAY'S OBJECTIVE: Introduce yourself (use a pleasant face and voice; look at the person; tell the person your name; ask for the person's name). When you introduce yourself you will know the person's name; you will seem friendlier; you will have more friends; people will like you because you are polite.

TARGET BEHAVIORS: In addition to introducing yourself, the following individual skills were practiced.

	Score	**Scale**
A. _____	____	1 = completely satisfied
B. _____	____	2 = satisfied
		3 = slightly satisfied
C. _____	____	4 = neither satisfied nor dissatisfied
D. _____	____	5 = slightly dissatisfied
		6 = dissatisfied
E. _____	____	7 = completely dissatisfied

The best thing done today: _____

_____

✂ —

PLEASE COMPLETE THIS SECTION AND RETURN

Client Name _____

SKILL 6: Introduce yourself

Did the participant use today's skill at least once this week?

	Yes	No
1. Use a pleasant face and voice.	____	____
2. Look at the person.	____	____
3. Tell the person your name.	____	____
4. Ask for the person's name.	____	____

TARGET BEHAVIORS: Use the 1–7 scale to rate the target behaviors listed above.

COMMENTS:

A. ____
B. ____
C. ____
D. ____
E. ____

Signature _____ Date _____

Homework

Client Name _____ Date _____

1. What are four things you can do or say to introduce yourself to someone you don't know?

   a. _____

   b. _____

   c. _____

   d. _____

2. Before the next group, introduce yourself to at least one new person.

   a. Where were you? _____

   b. Whom did you meet? _____

   c. What did you say? _____

   _____

   d. What did the other person do or say? _____

   _____

Skill 7: Give Positive Feedback

Follow the instructions provided in Session Outline 2 for conducting • Conversation Time and Homework Completion and • Relaxation Training. Then go on to the • Skill Lesson.

SKILL LESSON

Introduce skill and list components.

Instructor 1: *(Ask participants to form a circle.)* Today we are going to talk about how to give positive feedback. To give positive feedback, you:

- Use a pleasant face and voice.

- Look at the person.

- Tell the person something good about what he or she did.

- Tell the person right away.

Role-play appropriate example.

Instructor 1: This is the right way to give positive feedback. I'm with (Instructor 2), who has just brought me back from bowling. Thanks, (Instructor 2), that was nice of you to bring me home!

Instructor 2: Sure, you're welcome.

Ask participants for skill components.

Instructor 1: How did you know that was the right way to give positive feedback? *(Participants respond or are prompted.)*

Role-play inappropriate example.

Instructor 1: This is the wrong way to give positive feedback. I'm with (Instructor 2), who has just brought me back from bowling. (No eye contact, but with pleasant face and voice) 'Bye, (Instructor 2).

Instructor 2: Goodbye.

Ask participants for skill components.

Instructor 1: What should have happened to make that the right way to give positive feedback? *(Participants respond or are prompted.)*

Ask participants to role-play.

Instructor 1: Now it's your turn to role-play. I am going to call on someone who has been working really hard in the group today by (name specific on-task behaviors). _____ has been (name appropriate behaviors) and looks ready to be the first one to role-play. _____, this is your role-play.

(Describe the role-play you have previously selected for this participant from the role-play chart following this session outline. Have each participant role-play the skill correctly at least once, using a previously selected situation.)

Ask participants to give positive feedback.

Instructor 1 or 2: Good role-playing. Who can tell _____ what he/she did right to give positive feedback in the role-play? *(Call on a participant who is volunteering and paying attention.)*

Ask participants for rationales for using skill.

Instructor 1: Why do you think it is important to give positive feedback? *(Participants respond or are prompted.)*

Possible responses:

- It makes people feel important or good.

- It makes friends.

- It helps people want to do well more often.

- It makes people happier to do things for you.

Lead participants through reality check.

Instructor 1: Sometimes you try really hard to give positive feedback, and this might happen. I'm with (Instructor 2), who has just brought me back from bowling. Thanks, (Instructor 2), that was nice of you to bring me home!

Instructor 2: You'd better thank me! I have a lot of things to do today, and bringing you here really messes up my schedule!

Instructor 1: You just did everything right to give positive feedback. What should you do if this happens to you? *(Participants respond or are prompted.)*

Possible responses:

- Take a deep breath to get calm.

- Show a good attitude.

- Ignore.

- Try again later.

Follow the instructions provided in Session Outline 2 for conducting • Refreshment Time • Activity • Home Notes and • New Homework.

Suggested activities for Session 7: Directed Drawing, Draw a Town—see Appendix B.

Role-Plays

Home

You can't find the blouse you wanted to wear today. Your roommate offers to help you look for it.

You are having trouble with the new washer. Your friend offers to show you how to run it.

You want to watch a new TV program. Your brother is watching another show. He offers to let you see your program.

Your dad is wearing the new tie you gave him. You think he looks nice.

Community

When you get to the store, you find out you don't have enough money. Your friend lends you the money.

You lost your purse. A woman calls you to say she found it on the bus.

You get to the movies late, and your friend is waiting for you.

A new person at bowling offers to let you use her ball.

Work

Your friend invites you to go out after work with another coworker.

Your supervisor lets you be first to try a new job.

Your friend comes to work with a new haircut.

You are having trouble finishing your work. Your coworker offers to help you so you can go on break.

School

Your teacher spends extra time with you on your assignment.

A bunch of people are playing softball, and they say you can join them.

You are having trouble with your homework, and your friend offers to help you.

Your teacher is sick, and the substitute does a good job of explaining the lesson.

Home Note

Client Name _____ Date _____

TODAY'S OBJECTIVE: Give positive feedback (use a pleasant face and voice; look at the person; tell the person something good about what he or she did; tell the person right away). When you give positive feedback it makes people feel important or good; it makes friends; it helps people want to do well more often; it makes people happier to do things for you.

TARGET BEHAVIORS: In addition to giving positive feedback, the following individual skills were practiced.

		Score	**Scale**
A.	_____	_____	1 = completely satisfied
B.	_____	_____	2 = satisfied
			3 = slightly satisfied
C.	_____	_____	4 = neither satisfied nor dissatisfied
D.	_____	_____	5 = slightly dissatisfied
			6 = dissatisfied
E.	_____	_____	7 = completely dissatisfied

The best thing done today: _____

_____

✂ —

PLEASE COMPLETE THIS SECTION AND RETURN

Client Name _____

SKILL 7: Give positive feedback

Did the participant use today's skill at least once this week?

	Yes	No
1. Use a pleasant face and voice.	____	____
2. Look at the person.	____	____
3. Tell the person something good about what he or she did.	____	____
4. Tell the person right away.	____	____

TARGET BEHAVIORS: Use the 1–7 scale to rate the target behaviors listed above.

COMMENTS:

A. ____

B. ____

C. ____

D. ____

E. ____

Signature _____ Date _____

Homework

Client Name _____ Date _____

1. Give positive feedback to someone you live with.

    a. What did you say? _____

    _____

    _____

    b. What did the other person say? _____

    _____

    _____

2. Draw a picture of someone giving positive feedback.

Skill 8: Accept Positive Feedback

> Follow the instructions provided in Session Outline 2 for conducting • Conversation Time and Homework Completion and • Relaxation Training. Then go on to the • Skill Lesson.

SKILL LESSON

Introduce skill and list components.

Instructor 1: *(Ask participants to form a circle.)* Today we are going to talk about how to accept positive feedback. To accept positive feedback, you:

- Use a pleasant face and voice.
- Look at the person.
- Listen to what the person says.
- Acknowledge the feedback by saying, "Thank you."

Role-play appropriate example.

Instructor 1: This is the right way to accept positive feedback. My teacher is giving me back an assignment.

Instructor 2: (Instructor 1), you did a great job on that math paper; every answer was correct!

Instructor 1: (Uses pleasant face and voice, looks at Instructor 2.) Thank you.

Ask participants for skill components.

Instructor 1: How did you know that was the right way to accept positive feedback? *(Participants respond or are prompted.)*

Role-play inappropriate example.

Instructor 1: This is the wrong way to accept positive feedback. My teacher is giving me back an assignment.

Instructor 2: (Instructor 1), you did a great job on that math paper; every answer was correct!

Instructor 1: (Looks down, blank face.) I didn't do the next assignment very well.

Ask participants for skill components.

Instructor 1: What should have happened to make that the right way to accept positive feedback? *(Participants respond or are prompted.)*

Ask participants to role-play.

Instructor 1: Now it's your turn to role-play. I am going to call on someone who has been working really hard in the group today by (name specific on-task behaviors). _____ has been (name appropriate behaviors) and looks ready to be the first one to role-play. _____, this is your role-play.

(Describe the role-play you have previously selected for this participant from the role-play chart following this session outline. Have each participant role-play the skill correctly at least once, using a previously selected situation.)

Ask participants to give positive feedback.

Instructor 1 or 2: Good role-playing. Who can tell _____ what he/she did right to accept positive feedback in the role-play? *(Call on a participant who is volunteering and paying attention.)*

Ask participants for rationales for using skill.

Instructor 1: Why do you think it is important to accept positive feedback? *(Participants respond or are prompted.)*

Possible responses:

- You will get more compliments.
- People will like you.
- You will feel good about yourself.
- People will know you feel good about yourself.

Lead participants through reality check.

Instructor 1: Sometimes you try really hard to accept positive feedback, and this might happen. My teacher is giving me back an assignment.

Instructor 2: (Instructor 1), you did a great job on that math paper; every answer was correct!

Instructor 1: (Uses pleasant face and voice, looks at the teacher.) Thank you.

Instructor 2: Well, now, you could show a little more enthusiasm, don't you think?

Instructor 1: You just did everything right to accept positive feedback. What should you do if this happens to you? *(Participants respond or are prompted.)*

Possible responses:

- Take a deep breath to get calm.

- Show a good attitude.

- Feel good about what you did.

- Say, "OK."

Follow the instructions provided in Session Outline 2 for conducting • Refreshment Time • Activity • Home Notes and • New Homework.

Suggested activity for Session 8: Draw a Town—see Appendix B.

Role-Plays

Home

Your roommate thanks you for not playing your radio too loudly.

Your dad thanks you for finishing your chore right away.

Your roommate compliments you on your new haircut.

Your brother or sister says, "Your room sure is clean!"

Community

The bus driver thanks you for staying so calm on the bus today.

A neighbor you know tells you how much she appreciates your sweeping her walk.

Someone at Special Olympics tells you your softball throw was real good.

The clerk at the store you go to a lot says you are a careful shopper.

Work

Your coworker compliments you on how fast you did your work today.

A friend says she really likes your shirt.

Your supervisor tells you, in front of others, that you made zero errors yesterday.

Someone compliments you on the lunch you made.

School

Your teacher is answering your question about the homework. She says you're doing a good job on it.

Students are choosing sides for a game. When you're chosen they say, "He/she is really good!"

On the way home another student says she likes you.

Someone you really like asks you to sit by him because you're nice.

SKILL 8: ACCEPT POSITIVE FEEDBACK # Home Note

Client Name _____ Date _____

TODAY'S OBJECTIVE: Accept positive feedback (use a pleasant face and voice; look at the person; listen to what the person says; acknowledge the feedback by saying, "Thank you"). When you accept positive feedback you will get more compliments; people will like you; you will feel good about yourself; people will know you feel good about yourself.

TARGET BEHAVIORS: In addition to accepting positive feedback, the following individual skills were practiced.

	Score	Scale

A. _____ _____   1 = completely satisfied

B. _____ _____   2 = satisfied
                                      3 = slightly satisfied

C. _____ _____   4 = neither satisfied nor dissatisfied

D. _____ _____   5 = slightly dissatisfied
                                      6 = dissatisfied

E. _____ _____   7 = completely dissatisfied

The best thing done today: _____

_____

✂ —

PLEASE COMPLETE THIS SECTION AND RETURN

Client Name _____

SKILL 8: Accept positive feedback

Did the participant use today's skill at least once this week?

	Yes	No
1. Use a pleasant face and voice.	___	___
2. Look at the person.	___	___
3. Listen to what the person says.	___	___
4. Acknowledge the feedback by saying, "Thank you."	___	___

TARGET BEHAVIORS: Use the 1–7 scale to rate the target behaviors listed above.

COMMENTS:

A. _____
B. _____
C. _____
D. _____
E. _____

Signature _____ Date _____

Homework

Client Name _____ Date _____

1. When someone gives you positive feedback, what should you do and say?

_____

_____

_____

_____

_____

2. What might happen if you forget to accept positive feedback the right way?

_____

_____

_____

_____

_____

3. Write down some positive feedback someone gave you. Write down exactly what the person said. How did it make you feel?

_____

_____

_____

_____

_____

Skill 9: Interrupt the Right Way

Follow the instructions provided in Session Outline 2 for conducting • Conversation Time and Homework Completion and • Relaxation Training. Then go on to the • Skill Lesson.

SKILL LESSON

Introduce skill and list components.

Instructor 1: *(Ask participants to form a circle.)* Today we are going to talk about how to interrupt the right way. To interrupt the right way, you:

- Use a pleasant face and voice.
- Wait for a pause.
- Look at the person.
- Say, "Excuse me."
- Wait until the person looks at you.

Role-play appropriate example.

Instructor 1: This is the right way to interrupt. I'm in the hallway, wearing my new Special Olympics medal. (Instructor 2) is talking to (a participant).

Instructor 2: (Talks with participant while Instructor 1 waits; there is a pause in the conversation.)

Instructor 1: (Uses pleasant face and voice, looks at Instructor 2.) Excuse me, (Instructor 2). I wanted to show you my Special Olympics medal.

Ask participants for skill components.

Instructor 1: How did you know that was the right way to interrupt? *(Participants respond or are prompted.)*

Role-play inappropriate example.

Instructor 1: This is the wrong way to interrupt. I'm in the hallway, wearing my new Special Olympics medal. (Instructor 2) is talking to (a participant).

Instructor 2: (Talks with participant while Instructor 1 approaches.)

Instructor 1: (Doesn't wait for a pause.) Hey, look, you guys, I got third place.

Ask participants for skill components.

Instructor 1: What should have happened to make that the right way to interrupt? (*Participants respond or are prompted.*)

Ask participants to role-play.

Instructor 1: Now it's your turn to role-play. I am going to call on someone who has been working really hard in the group today by (name specific on-task behaviors). _____ has been (name appropriate behaviors) and looks ready to be the first one to role-play. _____, this is your role-play.

(*Describe the role-play you have previously selected for this participant from the role-play chart following this session outline. Have each participant role-play the skill correctly at least once, using a previously selected situation.*)

Ask participants to give positive feedback.

Instructor 1 or 2: Good role-playing. Who can tell _____ what he/she did to interrupt the right way in the role-play? (*Call on a participant who is volunteering and paying attention.*)

Ask participants for rationales for using skill.

Instructor 1: Why do you think it is important to interrupt the right way? (*Participants respond or are prompted.*)

Possible responses:

- It helps you communicate better.

- People will want to listen to you.

- People will like you because you are polite.

Lead participants through reality check.

Instructor 1: Sometimes you try really hard to interrupt the right way, and this might happen. I'm in the hallway, wearing my new Special Olympics medal. (Instructor 2) is talking to (a participant).

Instructor 2: (Talks with participant while Instructor 1 waits; there is a pause in the conversation.)

Instructor 1: (Uses pleasant face and voice, looks at Instructor 2.) Excuse me, (Instructor 2). I wanted to show you my Special Olympics medal.

Instructor 2: Can't you see I'm busy? You're always interrupting!

Instructor 1: You just did everything right to interrupt correctly. What should you do if this happens to you? *(Participants respond or are prompted.)*

Possible responses:

- Take a deep breath to get calm.

- Show a good attitude.

- Ignore.

- Try again later.

Follow the instructions provided in Session Outline 2 for conducting • Refreshment Time • Activity • Home Notes and • New Homework.

Suggested activity for Session 9: Keeping Score—see Appendix B.

Role-Plays

Home

Your mom is talking to your brother. You need to tell her the vacuum cleaner isn't working.

Your roommates are talking about how to split up the housework this weekend. You already cleaned the bathrooms.

The apartment supervisor is talking to your roommate; you need to tell her you got in trouble at school today.

A couple of the others in your group home are talking about going swimming tomorrow; you want to ask if they've seen your brush.

Community

You need to ask a sales clerk where the men's clothes are. She is helping another customer.

You left your seat at the movie to get popcorn. Now the two people in the seats by the aisle are talking, and you want to get by.

Two women are talking together at the bus stop, and one of them drops something. You want to tell her about it before the bus comes.

At ski practice you get separated from your group. You need to ask directions; two coaches are standing nearby, talking.

Work

Your supervisor is giving instructions to a coworker. You want to go on a break now.

You're looking for a place to sit in the cafeteria. There is an empty spot next to two coworkers who are talking.

You forgot the next step in the job you are doing. Your supervisor is giving a tour to some people.

You are on a break and want to tell two coworkers about a movie you saw. They are talking about going to a party.

School

Your teacher is talking to another teacher in the lunch room. You want to tell her you lost your notebook.

You need some help with the reading assignment. The teacher is talking to another student.

Your teacher checks your work and says you can leave; you want to tell her you aren't finished, but she's talking to someone else.

Your friend is borrowing your book and talking to someone else. You need to tell him you need it before noon.

Home Note

Client Name _____ Date _____

TODAY'S OBJECTIVE: Interrupt the right way (use a pleasant face and voice; wait for a pause; look at the person; say, "Excuse me"; wait until the person looks at you). When you interrupt the right way it helps you communicate better; people will want to listen to you; people will like you because you are polite.

TARGET BEHAVIORS: In addition to interrupting the right way, the following individual skills were practiced.

	Score	Scale
A. _____	____	1 = completely satisfied
B. _____	____	2 = satisfied
		3 = slightly satisfied
C. _____	____	4 = neither satisfied nor dissatisfied
D. _____	____	5 = slightly dissatisfied
		6 = dissatisfied
E. _____	____	7 = completely dissatisfied

The best thing done today: _____

_____

✂ –

PLEASE COMPLETE THIS SECTION AND RETURN

Client Name _____

SKILL 9: Interrupt the right way

Did the participant use today's skill at least once this week?

	Yes	No
1. Use a pleasant face and voice.	____	____
2. Wait for a pause.	____	____
3. Look at the person.	____	____
4. Say, "Excuse me."	____	____
5. Wait until the person looks at you.	____	____

TARGET BEHAVIORS: Use the 1–7 scale to rate the target behaviors listed above.

COMMENTS:

A. ____

B. ____

C. ____

D. ____

E. ____

Signature _____ Date _____

Homework

Client Name _____ Date _____

1. Practice interrupting a conversation the right way:

   a. Use a pleasant face and voice.

   b. Wait for a pause.

   c. Look at the person.

   d. Say, "Excuse me."

   e. Wait until the person looks at you.

2. Interrupt another conversation the right way.

   a. Did you wait for a pause?

   (Circle one)   Yes   No

   b. What did you say? _____

   _____

   _____

Skill 10: Join in

> Follow the instructions provided in Session Outline 2 for conducting • Conversation Time and Homework Completion and • Relaxation Training. Then go on to the • Skill Lesson.

SKILL LESSON

Introduce skill and list components.

Instructor 1: *(Ask participants to form a circle.)* Today we are going to talk about joining in. To join in, you:

- Use a pleasant face and voice.
- Look at the person.
- Wait for a pause.
- Say something on the topic.

Role-play appropriate example.

Instructor 1: This is the right way to join in. My friend, (Instructor 2), is talking to (a participant) about a movie they saw.

Instructor 2: (Talks with participant while Instructor 1 waits; there is a pause in the conversation.)

Instructor 1: (Waits calmly for pause, then says something on the topic.) That movie you went to sure must have been interesting.

Ask participants for skill components.

Instructor 1: How did you know that was the right way to join in? *(Participants respond or are prompted.)*

Role-play inappropriate example.

Instructor 1: This is the wrong way to join in. My friend, (Instructor 2), is talking to (a participant) about a movie they saw.

Instructor 2: (Talks with participant.)

Instructor 1: (Doesn't wait for a pause; changes the subject.) Hey, Megan's going swimming with Kevin!

Ask participants for skill components.

Instructor 1: What should have happened to make that the right way to join in? *(Participants respond or are prompted.)*

Ask participants to role-play.

Instructor 1: Now it's your turn to role-play. I am going to call on someone who has been working really hard in the group today by (name specific on-task behaviors). _____ has been (name appropriate behaviors) and looks ready to be the first one to role-play. _____, this is your role-play.

(Describe the role-play you have previously selected for this participant from the role-play chart following this session outline. Have each participant role-play the skill correctly at least once, using a previously selected situation.)

Ask participants to give positive feedback.

Instructor 1 or 2: Good role-playing. Who can tell _____ what he/she did right to join in during the role-play? *(Call on a participant who is volunteering and paying attention.)*

Ask participants for rationales for using skill.

Instructor 1: Why do you think it is important to join in? *(Participants respond or are prompted.)*

Possible responses:

- People will listen to you more often.

- People will like you because you listened to them.

- It helps people hear what you have to say.

Lead participants through reality check.

Instructor 1: Sometimes you try really hard to join in, and this might happen. My friend, (Instructor 2), is talking to (a participant) about a movie they saw.

Instructor 2: (Talks with participant while Instructor 1 waits; there is a pause in the conversation.)

Instructor 1: (Waits calmly for a pause, then says something on the topic.) That movie you went to sure must have been interesting.

Instructor 2: Who cares what you think? Get lost!

Instructor 1: You just did everything right to join in. What should you do if this happens to you? *(Participants respond or are prompted.)*

114

Possible responses:

- Take a deep breath to get calm.

- Show a good attitude.

- Walk away.

- Go find someone else to talk to.

- Try again later.

Follow the instructions provided in Session Outline 2 for conducting • Refreshment Time • Activity • Home Notes and • New Homework.

Suggested activities for Session 10: Keeping Score, "Yes and . . ." —see Appendix B.

Role-Plays

Home

Some of the residents at the group home are planning a party.

Your mom is talking about how clean the kitchen is. You want to say your sister helped, too.

The group is deciding what the chore assignments will be for the week.

Your friends are talking about their day at work. You just got home, too.

Community

You are at the bus stop. Two people are trying to figure out which bus to take to the mall. You know which one.

You see the same people at the bus stop every day. They're talking to each other.

You're at basketball practice. The coach is talking to the group about a new shot. You want to try it.

You're at the restaurant with your friends. They're talking about plans for the upcoming holiday.

Work

Your supervisor is telling your coworker how to do a task. You have problems with that task, too.

At break, everyone is talking about Special Olympics. You were there, too.

Your supervisor is complimenting your friend on her work. You saw what a good job she did, too.

After lunch, two of your coworkers are helping to clean up the lunch room.

School

The teacher is showing your friend how to do the backstroke. You need to learn how, too.

Some classmates are talking about a new student. He shared his lunch with you.

The class got in trouble, and your teacher asks about how to have good behavior. You have an answer.

Your class is deciding what Christmas decorations to make for the classroom.

Home Note

Client Name _____ Date _____

TODAY'S OBJECTIVE: Join in (use a pleasant face and voice; look at the person; wait for a pause; say something on the topic). When you join in people will listen to you more often; people will like you because you listened to them; it helps people hear what you have to say.

TARGET BEHAVIORS: In addition to joining in, the following individual skills were practiced.

	Score	**Scale**
A. _____	_____	1 = completely satisfied
B. _____	_____	2 = satisfied
		3 = slightly satisfied
C. _____	_____	4 = neither satisfied nor dissatisfied
D. _____	_____	5 = slightly dissatisfied
		6 = dissatisfied
E. _____	_____	7 = completely dissatisfied

The best thing done today: _____

_____

✂ –

PLEASE COMPLETE THIS SECTION AND RETURN

Client Name _____

SKILL 10: Join in

Did the participant use today's skill at least once this week?

	Yes	No
1. Use a pleasant face and voice.	____	____
2. Look at the person.	____	____
3. Wait for a pause.	____	____
4. Say something on the topic.	____	____

TARGET BEHAVIORS: Use the 1–7 scale to rate the target behaviors listed above.

COMMENTS:

A. _____

B. _____

C. _____

D. _____

E. _____

Signature _____ Date _____

117

Homework

Client Name _____ Date _____

1. Go up to two or more people who are talking and join in their conversation. What are three things you remembered to do before you started talking?

   a. _____

   b. _____

   c. _____

2. Describe the conversation.

   a. What was the conversation about? _____

   _____

   b. What did you say? _____

   _____

3. Give two reasons why it is important to join a conversation the right way.

   a. _____

   b. _____

4. Name two things you could do if you tried to join a conversation the right way but were ignored.

   a. _____

   b. _____

Skill 11: Ignore

> Follow the instructions provided in Session Outline 2 for conducting • Conversation Time and Homework Completion and • Relaxation Training. Then go on to the • Skill Lesson.

SKILL LESSON

Introduce skill and list components.

Instructor 1: *(Ask participants to form a circle.)* Today we are going to talk about how to ignore. To ignore, you:

- Take a deep breath to get calm.
- Do not look at the person.
- Do not talk to the person.
- Walk away from the person if you can.

Role-play appropriate example.

Instructor 1: This is the right way to ignore. I'm at work, and my friend wants to talk. I need to do my job. (Keeps eyes on work during entire role-play.)

Instructor 2: (Taps Instructor 1 on the shoulder repeatedly.) Hey, (Instructor 1). Psst! (Eventually quits.)

Ask participants for skill components.

Instructor 1: How did you know that was the right way to ignore? *(Participants respond or are prompted.)*

Role-play inappropriate example.

Instructor 1: This is the wrong way to ignore. I'm at work, and my friend wants to talk. I need to do my job. (Keeps eyes on work.)

Instructor 2: (Taps Instructor 1 on the shoulder repeatedly.) Hey, (Instructor 1). Psst!

Instructor 1: (Looks at Instructor 2.) Sh-sh. Leave me alone. I'm trying to work.

Ask participants for skill components.

Instructor 1: What should have happened to make that the right way to ignore? *(Participants respond or are prompted.)*

Ask participants to role-play.

Instructor 1: Now it's your turn to role-play. I am going to call on someone who has been working really hard in the group today by (name specific on-task behaviors). _____ has been (name appropriate behaviors) and looks ready to be the first one to role-play. _____, this is your role-play.

(Describe the role-play you have previously selected for this participant from the role-play chart following this session outline. Have each participant role-play the skill correctly at least once, using a previously selected situation.)

Ask participants to give positive feedback.

Instructor 1 or 2: Good role-playing. Who can tell _____ what he/she did right to ignore in the role-play? *(Call on a participant who is volunteering and paying attention.)*

Ask participants for rationales for using skill.

Instructor 1: Why do you think it is important to ignore sometimes? *(Participants respond or are prompted.)*

Possible responses:

- It helps you keep out of trouble.

- If you aren't bothered, the person will probably quit.

- You won't get angry.

Lead participants through reality check.

Instructor 1: Sometimes you try really hard to ignore, and this might happen. (A participant) is at work, and his/her friend wants to talk. (The participant) needs to do his/her job. I will be the supervisor.

Participant: (Keeps eyes on work.)

Instructor 2: (Taps participant on the shoulder repeatedly.) Hey, _____. Psst!

Participant: (Ignores the right way.)

Instructor 1: (Continues heckling.)

Instructor 2: You guys better get back to work!

Instructor 1: You just did everything right to ignore. What should you do if this happens to you? *(Participants respond or are prompted.)*

Possible responses:

- Take a deep breath to get calm.

- Show a good attitude.

- Keep ignoring.

- Keep working.

- Keep quiet.

Follow the instructions provided in Session Outline 2 for conducting • Refreshment Time • Activity • Home Notes and • New Homework.

Suggested activities for Session 11: Simon Says, Heroes and Villains, Teasing Game—see Appendix B.

Role-Plays

Home

It is bedtime. You turned off the light, and your roommate switched it back on.

Your mom asks your brother or sister to pick up. He/she whines at you, "It's not fair. You never do anything around here!"

As you clear the table, a housemate shoves you and says, "Don't drop the glasses, Butterfingers."

The phone rings, and you answer. No one talks on the other end; it sounds like breathing.

Community

A group of kids on the corner laugh and jeer at you as you walk by.

Some kids drive by you, cursing and honking the horn. You are crossing the street in a crosswalk.

A woman sitting on the sidewalk asks you for a quarter as you go by.

A group of boys whistle and hoot at you, saying, "Hey, sweet thing, come over here."

Work

A coworker says, "You're my best friend. I need $10.00. Please lend me the money."

The person working next to you wants to talk. He asks loudly why you won't talk.

Your supervisor is giving you instructions. Some other workers are talking and making faces behind the supervisor's back.

Some women at work are giggling and looking at you. One calls out to you, "Hey, handsome."

School

A friend wants you to go to the store during lunch. You are not supposed to leave the school grounds.

Some classmates want you to pass a note during class.

A group of girls stop talking and whisper as you walk by on your way to class.

You are reading out loud for the whole class. Someone laughs when you stumble over a word.

SKILL 11: IGNORE   # Home Note

Client Name _____ Date _____

TODAY'S OBJECTIVE: Ignore (take a deep breath to get calm; do not look at the person; do not talk to the person; walk away from the person if you can). When you ignore it helps you keep out of trouble; if you aren't bothered, the person will probably quit; you won't get angry.

TARGET BEHAVIORS: In addition to ignoring, the following individual skills were practiced.

		Score	**Scale**
A.	_____	____	1 = completely satisfied
B.	_____	____	2 = satisfied
			3 = slightly satisfied
C.	_____	____	4 = neither satisfied nor dissatisfied
D.	_____	____	5 = slightly dissatisfied
			6 = dissatisfied
E.	_____	____	7 = completely dissatisfied

The best thing done today: _____

_____

✂ —

PLEASE COMPLETE THIS SECTION AND RETURN

Client Name _____

SKILL 11: Ignore

Did the participant use today's skill at least once this week?

	Yes	No
1. Take a deep breath to get calm.	____	____
2. Do not look at the person.	____	____
3. Do not talk to the person.	____	____
4. Walk away from the the person if you can.	____	____

TARGET BEHAVIORS: Use the 1–7 scale to rate the target behaviors listed above.

COMMENTS:

A. ____
B. ____
C. ____
D. ____
E. ____

Signature _____ Date _____

Homework

Client Name _____ Date _____

1. List two things you would do to ignore.

   a. _____

   b. _____

2. Name three examples of times when you would want to ignore someone.

   a. _____

   b. _____

   c. _____

3. Describe a time when you ignored.

   a. Who or what were you ignoring? _____

   b. What did you do? _____

   _____

   _____

   c. What happened? _____

   _____

   _____

4. If you ignore someone but the person keeps bothering you, what are three things you can do?

   a. _____

   b. _____

   c. _____

Skill 12: Accept No as an Answer

Follow the instructions provided in Session Outline 2 for conducting • Conversation Time and Homework Completion and • Relaxation Training. Then go on to the • Skill Lesson.

SKILL LESSON

Introduce skill and list components.

Instructor 1: *(Ask participants to form a circle.)* Today we are going to talk about how to accept no as an answer. To accept no as an answer, you:

- Use a pleasant face and voice.
- Take a deep breath to get calm.
- Look at the person.
- Say, "OK."
- Don't argue or make excuses.

Role-play appropriate example.

Instructor 1: This is the right way to accept no as an answer. My friends came over just before dinner and asked me to play basketball. (Instructor 2) is my home manager. (To Instructor 2) Can I go out and play basketball?

Instructor 2: No, it's almost time for dinner, and I want you to set the table.

Instructor 1: (Uses pleasant face and voice, takes a deep breath to get calm, looks at Instructor 2.) OK.

Ask participants for skill components.

Instructor 1: How did you know that was the right way to accept no as an answer? *(Participants respond or are prompted.)*

Role-play inappropriate example.

Instructor 1: This is the wrong way to accept no as an answer. My friends came over just before dinner and asked me to play basketball. (Instructor 2) is my home manager. (To Instructor 2) Can I go out and play basketball?

Instructor 2: No, it's almost time for dinner, and I want you to set the table.

Instructor 1: (Shows anger in face and voice.) Aw, come on. That's not fair! I just want to play for 5 minutes!

Ask participants for skill components.

Instructor 1: What should have happened to make that the right way to accept no as an answer? *(Participants respond or are prompted.)*

Ask participants to role-play.

Instructor 1: Now it's your turn to role-play. I am going to call on someone who has been working really hard in the group today by (name specific on-task behaviors). _____ has been (name appropriate behaviors) and looks ready to be the first one to role-play. _____, this is your role-play.

(Describe the role-play you have previously selected for this participant from the role-play chart following this session outline. Have each participant role-play the skill correctly at least once, using a previously selected situation.)

Ask participants to give positive feedback.

Instructor 1 or 2: Good role-playing. Who can tell _____ what he/she did right to accept no as an answer in the role-play? *(Call on a participant who is volunteering and paying attention.)*

Ask participants for rationales for using skill.

Instructor 1: Why do you think it is important to accept no as an answer? *(Participants respond or are prompted.)*

Possible responses:

- You won't get in trouble.

- You will earn more privileges.

- People will be happy with you.

Lead participants through reality check.

Instructor 1: Sometimes you try really hard to accept no as an answer, and this might happen. My friends came over just before dinner and asked me to play basketball. (Instructor 2) is my home manager. (To Instructor 2) Can I go out and play basketball?

Instructor 2: No, it's almost time for dinner, and I want you to set the table.

Instructor 1: (Uses pleasant face and voice, takes a deep breath to get calm, looks at Instructor 2.) OK.

Instructor 2: (Instructor 1), I don't like your attitude around here lately. I think you need to do some extra chores tonight.

Instructor 1: You just did everything right to accept no as an answer. What should you do if this happens to you? *(Participants respond or are prompted.)*

Possible responses:

- Take a deep breath to get calm.

- Keep a good attitude.

- Feel good about what you did.

- Say, "OK" and do what was asked.

Follow the instructions provided in Session Outline 2 for conducting • Refreshment Time • Activity • Home Notes and • New Homework.

Suggested activities for Session 12: "May I," Marble Game—see Appendix B.

Role-Plays

Home

You want to go over to your friend's house. Your mother says no because you need to clean your room.

You ask your roommate if you can wear her sweater today. She says no.

You want to have your own phone. Your father says no because it costs too much money.

You want to trade chores with your friend. Your group home manager says no.

Community

You want to be the first one at bowling. The supervisor says it's not your turn.

You want to try a new Mexican restaurant. Everyone else wants to have Chinese food tonight.

At the store you see a new tape you want. Your program supervisor says you need the money to do your laundry.

You're tired and want to take a taxi home. Your friend says to take the bus; a taxi is too expensive.

Work

You want to do a different job. Your supervisor tells you to keep working on the job you're doing.

You ask your friend to buy you a soft drink. He says he can't because he's buying Jane one.

You ask your supervisor to help you with a hard task. Your supervisor says she's too busy right now.

You ask if you can go to the bathroom. Your supervisor says to wait until break time.

School

You ask to help clean the chalkboards. Your teacher says it's Janice's turn.

You don't understand your math lesson, and you ask your teacher for help. He says you have to wait until later and to keep trying.

At lunch you want chocolate milk. The cafeteria staff tell you there's no more left.

You ask if you can bring your radio to school. Your teacher says no.

Home Note

Client Name _____ Date _____

TODAY'S OBJECTIVE: Accept no as an answer (use a pleasant face and voice; take a deep breath to get calm; look at the person; say, "OK"; don't argue or make excuses). When you accept no as an answer you won't get in trouble; you will earn more privileges; people will be happy with you.

TARGET BEHAVIORS: In addition to accepting no as an answer, the following individual skills were practiced.

	Score	Scale
A. _____ ____		1 = completely satisfied
B. _____ ____		2 = satisfied
		3 = slightly satisfied
C. _____ ____		4 = neither satisfied nor dissatisfied
D. _____ ____		5 = slightly dissatisfied
		6 = dissatisfied
E. _____ ____		7 = completely dissatisfied

The best thing done today: _____

_____

✂ –

PLEASE COMPLETE THIS SECTION AND RETURN

Client Name _____

SKILL 12: Accept no as an answer

Did the participant use today's skill at least once this week?

	Yes	No
1. Use a pleasant face and voice.	____	____
2. Take a deep breath to get calm.	____	____
3. Look at the person.	____	____
4. Say, "OK."	____	____
5. Don't argue or make excuses.	____	____

TARGET BEHAVIORS: Use the 1–7 scale to rate the target behaviors listed above.

COMMENTS:

A. ____

B. ____

C. ____

D. ____

E. ____

Signature _____ Date _____

Homework

Client Name _____ Date _____

1. Write down a time when someone said no to you about something you wanted.

    a. What happened? _____

    _____

    _____

    b. How did you feel? _____

    _____

    _____

    c. What did you do? _____

    _____

    _____

    d. What did the other person do? _____

    _____

    _____

2. Practice accepting no for an answer the right way. What are five things you did?

    a. _____

    b. _____

    c. _____

    d. _____

    e. _____

3. Name two reasons why it is important to accept no as an answer.

    a. _____

    b. _____

Skill 13: Ask, Don't Tell

Follow the instructions provided in Session Outline 2 for conducting • Conversation Time and Homework Completion and • Relaxation Training. Then go on to the • Skill Lesson.

SKILL LESSON

Introduce skill and list components.

Instructor 1: *(Ask participants to form a circle.)* Today we are going to talk about how to ask, not tell. To ask, not tell, you:

- Use a pleasant face and voice.

- Ask, using a question.

- Accept no as an answer.

Role-play appropriate example.

Instructor 1: This is the right way to ask, not tell. I'm playing a game with a friend, and he/she isn't playing correctly. (To Instructor 2, using a pleasant face and voice) Could we please check the rules? I think it's my turn now.

Instructor 2: OK.

Ask participants for skill components.

Instructor 1: How did you know that was the right way to ask, not tell? *(Participants respond or are prompted.)*

Role-play inappropriate example.

Instructor 1: This is the wrong way to ask, not tell. I'm playing a game with a friend, and he/she isn't playing correctly. (To Instructor 2, frowning and raising voice) Hey, it's my turn now! Give me the dice!

Ask participants for skill components.

Instructor 1: What should have happened to make that the right way to ask, not tell? *(Participants respond or are prompted.)*

Ask participants to role-play.

Instructor 1: Now it's your turn to role-play. I am going to call on someone who has been working really hard in the group today by (name specific on-task behaviors). _____ has been (name appropriate behaviors) and looks ready to be the first one to role-play. _____, this is your role-play.

(Describe the role-play you have previously selected for this participant from the role-play chart following this session outline. Have each participant role-play the skill correctly at least once, using a previously selected situation.)

Ask participants to give positive feedback.

Instructor 1 or 2: Good role-playing. Who can tell _____ what he/she did right to ask, not tell in the role-play? *(Call on a participant who is volunteering and paying attention.)*

Ask participants for rationales for using skill.

Instructor 1: Why do you think it is important to ask, not tell? *(Participants respond or are prompted.)*

Possible responses:

- People will want to do what you want more often.

- People will enjoy doing things with you.

- People will like you.

Lead participants through reality check.

Instructor 1: Sometimes you try really hard to ask, not tell, and this might happen. I'm playing a game with a friend, and he/she isn't playing correctly. (To Instructor 2, using a pleasant face and voice) Could we please check the rules? I think it's my turn now.

Instructor 2: No, you're wrong; it's still my turn.

Instructor 1: You just did everything right to ask, not tell. What should you do if this happens to you? *(Participants respond or are prompted.)*

Possible responses:

- Take a deep breath to get calm.

- Show a good attitude.

- Feel good about what you did.

- Accept no as an answer.

Follow the instructions provided in Session Outline 2 for conducting • Refreshment Time • Activity • Home Notes and • New Homework.

Suggested activities for Session 13: Board Games, Draw a Town—see Appendix B.

Role-Plays

Home

You're talking about your day with staff when a housemate interrupts to show you his work note.

Your roommate borrowed your shampoo and has not returned it.

Your roommate is setting the table and puts the fork on the wrong side.

You are playing checkers with your sister. She does something you think is against the rules.

Community

You are out to dinner. The person next to you ordered french fries, and you'd like to taste one.

You overhear two people on the bus wondering where a store is. You know exactly where it is.

At bowling, someone picks up your ball to use.

You want to sit next to your friend on the bus, but someone is already sitting there.

Work

You've been really helpful to the person working next to you. Now you need help.

A coworker says you did your job all wrong. You just finished it.

You and a coworker made a big mess. Your boss tells only you to clean it up.

You want to make a phone call on your break, but someone is already using the phone.

School

Your pencil just broke. Your classmate has a new pen you want to borrow.

Your class is playing soccer. Some people on your team are not following the rules.

Someone cuts in ahead of you in the lunch line.

Two of you are working on a project. You have 10 minutes left to finish, but your partner is working really slowly.

Home Note

Client Name _____ Date _____

TODAY'S OBJECTIVE: Ask, don't tell (use a pleasant face and voice; ask, using a question; accept no as an answer). When you ask, don't tell, people will want to do what you want more often; people will enjoy doing things with you; people will like you.

TARGET BEHAVIORS: In addition to ask, don't tell, the following individual skills were practiced.

	Score	Scale
A. _____	____	1 = completely satisfied
B. _____	____	2 = satisfied
		3 = slightly satisfied
C. _____	____	4 = neither satisfied nor dissatisfied
D. _____	____	5 = slightly dissatisfied
		6 = dissatisfied
E. _____	____	7 = completely dissatisfied

The best thing done today: _____

_____

✂ –

PLEASE COMPLETE THIS SECTION AND RETURN

Client Name _____

SKILL 13: Ask, don't tell

Did the participant use today's skill at least once this week?

	Yes	No
1. Use a pleasant face and voice.	____	____
2. Ask, using a question.	____	____
3. Accept no as an answer.	____	____

TARGET BEHAVIORS: Use the 1–7 scale to rate the target behaviors listed above.

COMMENTS:

A. ____
B. ____
C. ____
D. ____
E. ____

Signature _____ Date _____

Homework

Client Name _____ Date _____

1. Write down a time when someone told you what to do.

    a. What happened? _____

    _____

    b. What did the person say? _____

    _____

    c. How did you feel? _____

    _____

2. Why is it important to ask instead of telling?

    _____

    _____

    _____

    _____

    _____

3. Write down a time when you asked for something at home.

    a. What did you say? _____

    _____

    b. What happened? _____

    _____

Skill 14: Solve Problems

Follow the instructions provided in Session Outline 2 for conducting • Conversation Time and Homework Completion and • Relaxation Training. Then go on to the • Skill Lesson.

SKILL LESSON

Introduce skill and list components.

Instructor 1: *(Ask participants to form a circle.)* Today we are going to talk about how to solve problems. To solve problems, you:

- Take a deep breath to get calm.

- Keep a good attitude.

- Think of at least one thing you can do.

- Try the best one.

Role-play appropriate example.

Instructor 1: This is the right way to solve problems. I'm at the bus stop, and I realize I forgot my lunch. The bus is coming in 10 minutes. I'm going to say what I'm thinking out loud so you can hear me. (Aloud to self) I sure am upset. What can I do? I'll take a deep breath to get calm, then I can think. I could run back to get my lunch. Or I could use my spending money to buy something to eat. Or I could ask someone to share lunch with me . . . I think I'll hurry back and get my lunch.

Ask participants for skill components.

Instructor 1: How did you know that was the right way to solve the problem? *(Participants respond or are prompted.)*

Role-play inappropriate example.

Instructor 1: This is the wrong way to solve problems. I'm at the bus stop, and I realize I forgot my lunch. The bus is coming in 10 minutes. (Aloud to self) I sure am upset. What can I do? I guess I just won't be able to go to work today.

Ask participants for skill components.

> Instructor 1: What should have happened to make that the right way to solve the problem? *(Participants respond or are prompted.)*

Ask participants to role-play.

> Instructor 1: Now it's your turn to role-play. I am going to call on someone who has been working really hard in the group today by (name specific on-task behaviors). _____ has been (name appropriate behaviors) and looks ready to be the first one to role-play. _____, this is your role-play.
>
> *(Describe the role-play you have previously selected for this participant from the role-play chart following this session outline. Have each participant role-play the skill correctly at least once, using a previously selected situation.)*

Ask participants to give positive feedback.

> Instructor 1 or 2: Good role-playing. Who can tell _____ what he/she did right to solve problems in the role-play? *(Call on a participant who is volunteering and paying attention.)*

Ask participants for rationales for using skill.

> Instructor 1: Why do you think it is important to solve problems? *(Participants respond or are prompted.)*
>
> Possible responses:
>
> - Things will go more smoothly.
>
> - You will get into less trouble.
>
> - You will feel better about yourself.
>
> - You will learn to be on your own (independent).

Lead participants through reality check.

> Instructor 1: Sometimes you try really hard to solve problems, and this might happen. I'm at the bus stop, and I realize I forgot my lunch. The bus is coming in 10 minutes. (Aloud to self) I sure am upset. What can I do? I'll take a deep breath to get calm, then I can think. I could run back to get my lunch. Or I could use my spending money to buy something to eat. Or I could ask someone to share lunch with me . . . I think I'll hurry back and get my lunch. (To participants) So I hurry back and get my lunch, but the bus comes a bit early and I miss it! You just did everything right to solve the problem. What should you do if this happens to you? *(Participants respond or are prompted.)*

Possible responses:

- Take a deep breath to get calm.

- Show a good attitude.

- Think of something you can do about your new problem.

Follow the instructions provided in Session Outline 2 for conducting • Refreshment Time • Activity • Home Notes and • New Homework.

Suggested activities for Session 14: Board Games, Problem Game—see Appendix B.

Role-Plays

Home

You are at a friend's, and you aren't sure what time you are supposed to be home.

You're eating dinner, and you don't like what was cooked.

Your roommate calls you a name. Just as you yell at her for it, a staff member walks in.

Your brother or sister is watching TV, and it is almost time for your favorite program.

Community

You're taking care of your neighbors' cat, and you can't remember where they said the key would be.

You're counting out change at the store. You don't have enough money.

You are at Special Olympics, and another athlete gets hurt just when it's your turn to compete.

As you get off the bus, you hurt your ankle. It hurts too much to walk home.

Work

When you get to work, someone else is doing the job your supervisor assigned to you yesterday.

The person next to you is bothering you. Your supervisor told you to deal with it.

At lunch, a friend gets mad at you because you won't give him half of your lunch.

You can't finish your assigned job because parts are missing. Your supervisor has left for an hour.

School

You get a C on your report card, but you think you deserved a better grade.

At lunch people are talking about skiing; you'd like to talk to them, but you don't know anything about skiing.

Another student asks you for some money so she can buy lunch. You have $3.00.

There's a substitute teacher in your class today. She thinks you should be able to do work that's too difficult for you.

Home Note

Client Name _____ Date _____

TODAY'S OBJECTIVE: Solve problems (take a deep breath to get calm; keep a good attitude; think of at least one thing you can do; try the best one). When you solve problems things will go more smoothly; you will get into less trouble; you will feel better about yourself; you will learn to be on your own (independent).

TARGET BEHAVIORS: In addition to solving problems, the following individual skills were practiced.

		Score	**Scale**
A.	_____	_____	1 = completely satisfied
B.	_____	_____	2 = satisfied
			3 = slightly satisfied
C.	_____	_____	4 = neither satisfied nor dissatisfied
D.	_____	_____	5 = slightly dissatisfied
			6 = dissatisfied
E.	_____	_____	7 = completely dissatisfied

The best thing done today: _____

_____

✂ –

PLEASE COMPLETE THIS SECTION AND RETURN

Client Name _____

SKILL 14: Solve problems

Did the participant use today's skill at least once this week?

	Yes	No
1. Take a deep breath to get calm.	____	____
2. Keep a good attitude.	____	____
3. Think of at least one thing you can do.	____	____
4. Try the best one.	____	____

TARGET BEHAVIORS: Use the 1–7 scale to rate the target behaviors listed above.

COMMENTS:

A. ____

B. ____

C. ____

D. ____

E. ____

Signature _____ Date _____

Homework

Client Name _____ Date _____

1. Write down a problem you had this week at home. How did you solve it?

   _____

   _____

   _____

   _____

   _____

   _____

   _____

2. Write down a problem you had this week somewhere besides home. How did you solve it?

   _____

   _____

   _____

   _____

   _____

   _____

   _____

Skill 15: Accept Consequences

> Follow the instructions provided in Session Outline 2 for conducting • Conversation Time and Homework Completion and • Relaxation Training. Then go on to the • Skill Lesson.

SKILL LESSON

Introduce skill and list components.

Instructor 1: *(Ask participants to form a circle.)* Today we are going to talk about how to accept consequences. To accept consequences, you:

- Take a deep breath to get calm.
- Use a pleasant face and voice.
- Listen to the person giving the consequence.
- Say, "OK."

Role-play appropriate example.

Instructor 1: This is the right way to accept consequences. I goofed off on the job, and my supervisor is giving me a consequence.

Instructor 2: OK, (Instructor 1). Thanks for paying attention to me right now. I need to talk to you about the break. You were playing around, and you were 15 minutes late coming back. I'm going to have to take off 5 points on your point card.

Instructor 1: (Takes a deep breath, keeps a pleasant face and voice, looks at Instructor 2.) OK.

Ask participants for skill components.

Instructor 1: How did you know that was the right way to accept consequences? *(Participants respond or are prompted.)*

Role-play inappropriate example.

Instructor 1: This is the wrong way to accept consequences. I goofed off on the job, and my supervisor is giving me a consequence.

Instructor 2: OK, (Instructor 1). Thanks for paying attention to me right now. I need to talk to you about the break. You were playing around, and you were 15 minutes late coming back. I'm going to have to take off 5 points on your point card.

Instructor 1: (Frowns, begins talking before Instructor 2 finishes.) That's not true—I was only a few minutes late. That's not fair; I need those points!

Ask participants for skill components.

Instructor 1: What should have happened to make that the right way to accept consequences? *(Participants respond or are prompted.)*

Ask participants to role-play.

Instructor 1: Now it's your turn to role-play. I am going to call on someone who has been working really hard in the group today by (name specific on-task behaviors). _____ has been (name appropriate behaviors) and looks ready to be the first one to role-play. _____, this is your role-play.

(Describe the role-play you have previously selected for this participant from the role-play chart following this session outline. Have each participant role-play the skill correctly at least once, using a previously selected situation.)

Ask participants to give positive feedback.

Instructor 1 or 2: Good role-playing. Who can tell _____ what he/she did right to accept consequences in the role-play? *(Call on a participant who is volunteering and paying attention.)*

Ask participants for rationales for using skill.

Instructor 1: Why do you think it is important to accept consequences? *(Participants respond or are prompted.)*

Possible responses:

- People will do more things for you.

- Things will go more smoothly.

- You won't get into more trouble.

Lead participants through reality check.

Instructor 1: Sometimes you try really hard to accept consequences, and this might happen. I goofed off on the job, and my supervisor is giving me a consequence.

Instructor 2: OK, (Instructor 1). Thanks for paying attention to me right now. I need to talk to you about the break. You were playing around, and you were 15 minutes late coming back. I'm going to have to take off 5 points on your point card.

Instructor 1: (Takes a deep breath, keeps a pleasant face, looks at Instructor 2.) OK.

Instructor 2: And if I catch you goofing off one more time, you've had it!

Instructor 1: You just did everything right to accept consequences. What should you do if this happens to you? *(Participants respond or are prompted.)*

Possible responses:

- Take a deep breath to get calm.

- Show a good attitude.

- Work hard at being on time.

Follow the instructions provided in Session Outline 2 for conducting • Refreshment Time • Activity • Home Notes and • New Homework.

Suggested activities for Session 15: Board Games, Marble Game—see Appendix B.

Role-Plays

Home

The group home operator offered to take you to the store but said she was leaving in 5 minutes. Now she's leaving, and you're not ready.

Everyone was talking about what movie to see. You didn't say which one you preferred, and now they've decided to go to one you don't want to see.

You were told that if you didn't do your chores you wouldn't be able to go on the Sunday outing. You only did half the chores.

Your job tonight is to do dishes; you watched TV all evening. Now it's late, and you're tired.

Community

You want to ride the bus home, but you spent all your money on soda pop. Now the bus driver says you can't get on if you don't have the money.

You and your friend are talking loudly and giggling during a movie. Now the theater manager is telling you to leave.

You walk all the way to the video store to get a movie. You didn't call first, and the store is closed when you get there.

You spent a long time at lunch and missed the bus.

Work

You were trying to get done early, so you skipped some steps. Your boss caught the mistakes and said you have to stay and redo your work.

Yesterday you were saying mean things about a coworker. Today she and her friends won't sit with you.

You thought your mom would buy some soda pop for you. She didn't, and now you don't have a drink in your lunch.

You were daydreaming, so you didn't get much work done. That means you'll have less money this week.

School

Your teacher set up a movie outing for those students who completed their reading project on time. You didn't.

You didn't do your homework, so now you have to stay in to do it.

Your teacher wants you to read out loud. You don't know where to start because you weren't listening.

You need two pencils for a test, but you only have one. The teacher says you can buy one with some of your points.

Home Note

Client Name _____ Date _____

TODAY'S OBJECTIVE: Accept consequences (take a deep breath to get calm; use a pleasant face and voice; listen to the person giving the consequence; say, "OK"). When you accept consequences people will do more things for you; things will go more smoothly; you won't get into more trouble.

TARGET BEHAVIORS: In addition to accepting consequences, the following individual skills were practiced.

	Score	**Scale**
A. _____	____	1 = completely satisfied
B. _____	____	2 = satisfied
		3 = slightly satisfied
C. _____	____	4 = neither satisfied nor dissatisfied
D. _____	____	5 = slightly dissatisfied
		6 = dissatisfied
E. _____	____	7 = completely dissatisfied

The best thing done today: _____

_____

✂ —

PLEASE COMPLETE THIS SECTION AND RETURN

Client Name _____

SKILL 15: Accept consequences

Did the participant use today's skill at least once this week?

	Yes	No
1. Take a deep breath to get calm.	____	____
2. Use a pleasant face and voice.	____	____
3. Listen to the person giving the consequence.	____	____
4. Say, "OK."	____	____

TARGET BEHAVIORS: Use the 1–7 scale to rate the target behaviors listed above.

COMMENTS:

A. ____

B. ____

C. ____

D. ____

E. ____

Signature _____ Date _____

Homework

Client Name _____ Date _____

1. Why is it important to take a deep breath when someone gives you a consequence?

   _____

   _____

   _____

   _____

2. Name two times when you accepted consequences.

   Time 1:

   a. What did the other person say? _____

   _____

   b. What did you do and say? _____

   _____

   Time 2:

   a. What did the other person say? _____

   _____

   b. What did you do and say? _____

   _____

3. Why is it a good idea to accept consequences the right way?

   _____

   _____

   _____

   _____

Skill 16: Take Responsibility

> Follow the instructions provided in Session Outline 2 for conducting • Conversation Time and Homework Completion and • Relaxation Training. Then go on to the • Skill Lesson.

SKILL LESSON

Introduce skill and list components.

Instructor 1: *(Ask participants to form a circle.)* Today we are going to talk about how to take responsibility. To take responsibility, you:

- Use a pleasant face and voice.
- Tell the truth.
- Make no excuses.
- Accept consequences with a good attitude.

Role-play appropriate example.

Instructor 1: This is the right way to take responsibility. My roommate works at another workshop, and I'm bored with mine. So I called in sick and went to work with my roommate, then spent the rest of the time downtown. (Instructor 2) is the supervisor at my apartment program, and he/she thinks something is wrong.

Instructor 2: (Instructor 1), were you at work today?

Instructor 1: No. I was goofing off.

Instructor 2: Well, I think you need to call your boss. And when you're through, I'd like to talk to you about this while the others are watching that special TV program.

Instructor 1: OK. I know I goofed up.

Ask participants for skill components.

Instructor 1: How did you know that was the right way to take responsibility? *(Participants respond or are prompted.)*

Role-play inappropriate example.

Instructor 1: This is the wrong way to take responsibility. My roommate works at another workshop, and I'm bored with mine. So I called in sick and went to work with my roommate, then spent the rest of the time downtown. (Instructor 2) is the supervisor at my apartment program, and he/she thinks something is wrong.

Instructor 2: (Instructor 1), were you at work today?

Instructor 1: I couldn't go because Jim made me go with him. He told me if I didn't, he wouldn't be my friend anymore.

Ask participants for skill components.

Instructor 1: What should have happened to make that the right way to take responsibility? *(Participants respond or are prompted.)*

Ask participants to role-play.

Instructor 1: Now it's your turn to role-play. I am going to call on someone who has been working really hard in the group today by (name specific on-task behaviors). _____ has been (name appropriate behaviors) and looks ready to be the first one to role-play. _____, this is your role-play.

(Describe the role-play you have previously selected for this participant from the role-play chart following this session outline. Have each participant role-play the skill correctly at least once, using a previously selected situation.)

Ask participants to give positive feedback.

Instructor 1 or 2: Good role-playing. Who can tell _____ what he/she did right to take responsibility in the role-play? *(Call on a participant who is volunteering and paying attention.)*

Ask participants for rationales for using skill.

Instructor 1: Why do you think it is important to take responsibility? *(Participants respond or are prompted.)*

Possible responses:

- You will get more things you want.

- People will believe what you say.

- You won't get into trouble.

Lead participants through reality check.

Instructor 1: Sometimes you try really hard to take responsibility, and this might happen. My roommate works at another workshop, and I'm bored with mine. So I called in sick and went to work with my roommate, then spent the rest of the time downtown. (Instructor 2) is the supervisor at my apartment program, and he/she thinks something is wrong.

Instructor 2: (Instructor 1), were you at work today?

Instructor 1: No. I was goofing off.

Instructor 2: Well, I think you need to call your boss. And when you're through, I'd like to talk to you about this while the others are watching that special TV program.

Instructor 1: OK. I know I goofed up.

Instructor 2: And if you do this again, you're going to be kicked out of here. You're really skating on thin ice!

Instructor 1: You just did everything right to take responsibility. What should you do if this happens to you? *(Participants respond or are prompted.)*

Possible responses:

- Take a deep breath to get calm.

- Show a good attitude.

- Start working on following the rules better.

Follow the instructions provided in Session Outline 2 for conducting • Refreshment Time • Activity • Home Notes and • New Homework.

Suggested activities for Session 16: Board Games, "May I," Problem Game—see Appendix B.

Role-Plays

Home

Your visit with friends lasted longer than it was supposed to. When you get home, your home manager is waiting up for you.

You borrow your sister's new sweater and get ink on it. You try to wash it, but it's ruined.

You spend all your money for the week on new clothes. Your home operator asks you for your share of the phone bill.

You hurt yourself falling off your bike. You get mad at Tom and tell a staff member that Tom hurt you. Later, your counselor asks you what happened.

Community

Your friend asks you to come over. You say you'll be right there. You go to the movies instead. The next day you see your friend at work.

You are playing ball with your friends. You throw the ball and break your neighbor's window. Your neighbor is coming home.

You borrow your friend's bowling ball but forget it when you leave the lanes. Your friend calls and says he needs his ball tonight.

You forgot to take enough bus fare to get home from shopping. The bus driver knows you.

Work

You are working on a job that you don't like. You make a lot of mistakes. Your supervisor is coming over to check your work.

At lunch your coworker asks if you want to leave and go downtown. You say yes. The next morning you see your supervisor.

You forgot to bring your lunch to work today. Your supervisor tells you it's time for lunch.

You oversleep and miss the bus. When you finally get to work, your supervisor asks you what happened.

School

You stayed up late watching a movie on TV and didn't do your homework. Your teacher asks you to hand in your homework.

Your friend is sick and asks you to bring her book home from school. You forget it. She asks you for the book.

Your classmate knows how to write better than you do. You copy her answers on the test. Later your teacher asks why you have the same answers.

Your friend tells you a secret and asks you not to tell anyone. You tell your friend Judy. Later, your friend asks you how Judy found out.

Home Note

Client Name _____ Date _____

TODAY'S OBJECTIVE: Take responsibility (use a pleasant face and voice; tell the truth; make no excuses; accept consequences with a good attitude). When you take responsibility you will get more things you want; people will believe what you say; you won't get into trouble.

TARGET BEHAVIORS: In addition to taking responsibility, the following individual skills were practiced.

	Score	**Scale**
A. _____	_____	1 = completely satisfied
B. _____	_____	2 = satisfied
		3 = slightly satisfied
C. _____	_____	4 = neither satisfied nor dissatisfied
D. _____	_____	5 = slightly dissatisfied
		6 = dissatisfied
E. _____	_____	7 = completely dissatisfied

The best thing done today: _____

_____

✂ —

PLEASE COMPLETE THIS SECTION AND RETURN

Client Name _____

SKILL 16: Take responsibility

Did the participant use today's skill at least once this week?

	Yes	No
1. Use a pleasant face and voice.	____	____
2. Tell the truth.	____	____
3. Make no excuses.	____	____
4. Accept consequences with a good attitude.	____	____

TARGET BEHAVIORS: Use the 1–7 scale to rate the target behaviors listed above.

COMMENTS:

A. ____
B. ____
C. ____
D. ____
E. ____

Signature _____ Date _____

Homework

Client Name _____ Date _____

1. Tell about a time this week when you took responsibility by telling the truth, making no excuses, and accepting consequences.

   _____

   _____

   _____

   _____

   _____

2. Tell about a time this week when you did not take responsibility. What could you have done to take responsibility?

   _____

   _____

   _____

   _____

   _____

3. Why is it a good idea to take responsibility?

   _____

   _____

   _____

   _____

   _____

Skill 17: Say No to Stay Out of Trouble

> Follow the instructions provided in Session Outline 2 for conducting • Conversation Time and Homework Completion and • Relaxation Training. Then go on to the • Skill Lesson.

SKILL LESSON

Introduce skill and list components.

Instructor 1: *(Ask participants to form a circle.)* Today we are going to talk about how to say no to stay out of trouble. To say no to stay out of trouble, you:

- Take a deep breath to get calm.
- Look at the person.
- Keep saying no.
- Suggest something else to do.
- If that doesn't work, ignore and walk away.

Role-play appropriate example.

Instructor 1: This is the right way to say no to stay out of trouble. I'm at the store after school with my friend. We have no money. I say, "I would really like some candy."

Instructor 2: Just pick some up. If you put it in your pocket, the clerk won't notice.

Instructor 1: (Takes a deep breath, looks at Instructor 2.) No way. I don't steal.

Instructor 2: Just put it in your pocket.

Instructor 1: No. I don't steal. Let's go to my house—I have candy there.

Instructor 2: Come on, Chicken!

Instructor 1: (Ignores and walks away.)

Ask participants for skill components.

> Instructor 1: How did you know that was the right way to say no to stay out of trouble? *(Participants respond or are prompted.)*

Role-play inappropriate example.

> Instructor 1: This is the wrong way to say no to stay out of trouble. I'm at the store after school with my friend. We have no money. I say, "I would really like some candy."

> Instructor 2: Just pick some up. If you put it in your pocket, the clerk won't notice.

> Instructor 1: (Takes a deep breath, looks at Instructor 2.) No way. I don't steal.

> Instructor 2: Just put it in your pocket.

> Instructor 1: Well . . . OK.

Ask participants for skill components.

> Instructor 1: What should have happened to make that the right way to say no to stay out of trouble? *(Participants respond or are prompted.)*

Ask participants to role-play.

> Instructor 1: Now it's your turn to role-play. I am going to call on someone who has been working really hard in the group today by (name specific on-task behaviors). _____ has been (name appropriate behaviors) and looks ready to be the first one to role-play. _____, this is your role-play.
>
> *(Describe the role-play you have previously selected for this participant from the role-play chart following this session outline. Have each participant role-play the skill correctly at least once, using a previously selected situation.)*

Ask participants to give positive feedback.

> Instructor 1 or 2: Good role-playing. Who can tell _____ what he/she did right to say no to stay out of trouble in the role-play? *(Call on a participant who is volunteering and paying attention.)*

Ask participants for rationales for using skill.

> Instructor 1: Why do you think it is important to say no to stay out of trouble? *(Participants respond or are prompted.)*
>
> Possible responses:
>
> • It keeps you out of trouble.

- You feel better for making your own decisions and choices.

- Others will trust you more.

- You take responsibility for yourself.

Lead participants through reality check.

Instructor 1: Sometimes you try really hard to say no to stay out of trouble, and this might happen. I'm at the store after school with my friend. We have no money. I say, "I would really like some candy."

Instructor 2: Just pick some up. If you put it in your pocket, the clerk won't notice.

Instructor 1: (Takes a deep breath, looks at Instructor 2.) No way. I don't steal.

Instructor 2: Just put it in your pocket.

Instructor 1: No. I don't steal. Let's go to my house—I have candy there.

Instructor 2: Come on, Chicken!

Instructor 1: (Ignores and walks away.)

Instructor 2: You're such a jerk. I'm never going to be your friend again.

Instructor 1: You just did everything right to say no to stay out of trouble. What should you do if this happens to you? *(Participants respond or are prompted.)*

Possible responses:

- Take a deep breath to get calm.

- Show a good attitude.

- Walk away.

- Ignore name-calling.

- Find someone else to spend time with.

Follow the instructions provided in Session Outline 2 for conducting • Refreshment Time • Activity • Home Notes and • New Homework.

Suggested activity for Session 17: Heroes and Villains—see Appendix B.

Role-Plays

Home

Your brother forgot to put his bike away and wants you to lie about it for him.

Your brother-in-law wants to try your medication. He is willing to pay you.

Your uncle asks if you need help getting dressed.

Your sister spent all her allowance. She wants you to ask your parents for yours and then give it to her.

Community

Your boyfriend wants to have sex without using a condom.

At the city bus center, a man asks you for money.

A stranger offers you a ride home. It's dark, and you're late.

Your friend wants you to buy a record, but you need all your money for groceries.

Work

One of your friends wants you to help play a joke on your boss by hiding his car keys.

A friend at work invites you to his apartment after work. You have an appointment.

Your best friend wants you to leave work at noon and go hang out downtown.

Your boyfriend lost his temper and got suspended from work. He wants you to skip work today and be with him.

School

Someone is giving out pills that she says will make you feel real good.

An older person wants to touch you. You two are the only ones in the bathroom.

While putting books away, you break a vase. Your friend says to hide the pieces and not tell the teacher.

Some guys will let you hang out with them if you'll go tell a girl you love her.

SKILL 17: SAY NO TO STAY OUT OF TROUBLE

Home Note

Client Name _____ Date _____

TODAY'S OBJECTIVE: Say no to stay out of trouble (take a deep breath to get calm; look at the person; keep saying no; suggest something else to do; if that doesn't work, ignore and walk away). When you say no it keeps you out of trouble; you feel better for making your own decisions and choices; others will trust you more; you take responsibility for yourself.

TARGET BEHAVIORS: In addition to saying no to stay out of trouble, the following individual skills were practiced.

	Score	Scale
A. _____	_____	1 = completely satisfied
B. _____	_____	2 = satisfied
		3 = slightly satisfied
C. _____	_____	4 = neither satisfied nor dissatisfied
D. _____	_____	5 = slightly dissatisfied
		6 = dissatisfied
E. _____	_____	7 = completely dissatisfied

The best thing done today: _____

_____

✂ —

PLEASE COMPLETE THIS SECTION AND RETURN

Client Name _____

SKILL 17: Say no to stay out of trouble

Did the participant use today's skill at least once this week?

	Yes	No
1. Take a deep breath to get calm.	____	____
2. Look at the person.	____	____
3. Keep saying no.	____	____
4. Suggest something else to do.	____	____
5. If that doesn't work, ignore and walk away.	____	____

TARGET BEHAVIORS: Use the 1-7 scale to rate the target behaviors listed above.

COMMENTS:

A. _____

B. _____

C. _____

D. _____

E. _____

Signature _____ Date _____

Homework

Client Name _____ Date _____

1. When someone asks you to do something you know is wrong, what are three things you can do?

   a. _____

   b. _____

   c. _____

2. This week, did someone ask you to do something you were not allowed to do?

   (Circle one)   Yes   No

3. If you answered yes to question 2, what happened?

   _____

   _____

   _____

   _____

   _____

Skill 18: Handle Name-Calling and Teasing

Follow the instructions provided in Session Outline 2 for conducting • Conversation Time and Homework Completion and • Relaxation Training. Then go on to the • Skill Lesson.

SKILL LESSON

Introduce skill and list components.

Instructor 1: *(Ask participants to form a circle.)* Today we are going to talk about how to handle name-calling and teasing. To handle name-calling and teasing, you:

- Take a deep breath to get calm.

- Keep a pleasant face.

- Look away or walk away if you can.

- Say nice things to yourself by thinking, I am calm; I can ignore.

Role-play appropriate example.

Instructor 1: This is the right way to handle name-calling and teasing. I'm at the bus stop, and a stranger is calling me names.

Instructor 2: Hey you! Why are you so funny looking? Are you dumb or something? You're the stupidest looking person I've ever seen.

Instructor 1: (Takes a deep breath, stays calm, looks away, maintains a pleasant face.) I'm thinking, I'm OK; I can keep calm; I can handle this.

Ask participants for skill components.

Instructor 1: How did you know that was the right way to handle name-calling and teasing? *(Participants respond or are prompted.)*

Role-play inappropriate example.

Instructor 1: This is the wrong way to handle name-calling and teasing. I'm at the bus stop, and a stranger is calling me names.

Instructor 2: Hey you! Why are you so funny looking? Are you dumb or something? You're the stupidest looking person I've ever seen.

Instructor 1: (Fidgets, gives eye contact, develops angry expression.) I am not stupid. Why don't you leave me alone!

Ask participants for skill components.

Instructor 1: What should have happened to make that the right way to handle name-calling and teasing? *(Participants respond or are prompted.)*

Ask participants to role-play.

Instructor 1: Now it's your turn to role-play. I am going to call on someone who has been working really hard in the group today by (name specific on-task behaviors). _____ has been (name appropriate behaviors) and looks ready to be the first one to role-play. _____, this is your role-play.

(Describe the role-play you have previously selected for this participant from the role-play chart following this session outline. Have each participant role-play the skill correctly at least once, using a previously selected situation.)

Ask participants to give positive feedback.

Instructor 1 or 2: Good role-playing. Who can tell _____ what he/she did right to handle name-calling and teasing in the role-play? *(Call on a participant who is volunteering and paying attention.)*

Ask participants for rationales for using skill.

Instructor 1: Why do you think it is important to handle name-calling and teasing? *(Participants respond or are prompted.)*

Possible responses:

- You will feel better about yourself.

- People will tease you less.

- You won't get in arguments or fights.

Lead participants through reality check.

Instructor 1: Sometimes you try really hard to handle name-calling and teasing, and this might happen. I'm at the bus stop, and a stranger is calling me names.

Instructor 2: Hey you! Why are you so funny looking? Are you dumb or something? You're the stupidest looking person I've ever seen.

Instructor 1: (Takes a deep breath, stays calm, looks away, maintains a pleasant face.) I'm thinking, I'm OK; I can keep calm; I can handle this.

Instructor 2: (Continues heckling.) Hey, I'm talking to you! Where did you get so dumb looking? You're not gonna ride my bus!

Instructor 1: You just did everything right to handle name-calling and teasing. What should you do if this happens to you? *(Participants respond or are prompted.)*

Possible responses:

- Take a deep breath to get calm.

- Show a good attitude.

- Keep ignoring.

- Walk away from the person.

- Find a different person to talk to.

Follow the instructions provided in Session Outline 2 for conducting • Refreshment Time • Activity • Home Notes and • New Homework.

Suggested activities for Session 18: Heroes and Villains, Teasing Game—see Appendix B.

Role-Plays

Home

Your roommate teases you about your girlfriend or boyfriend.

Your dad calls you "Slowpoke" as you're doing the dishes.

Your roommate teases you about your new haircut.

Your brother or sister says, "You're so stupid!"

Community

On the bus, some kids start pointing at you and calling you names.

You're counting out change at the store. The customer behind you says, "She sure is slow!"

Someone at Special Olympics makes fun of you for falling down.

While you're crossing the street, some guys in a car yell at you to hurry up.

Work

You put on makeup today and someone says, "You look like a clown."

Other workers are saying, "You're too slow."

A friend calls you a flirt because you were talking to your boyfriend or girlfriend.

Someone makes fun of the lunch that you made.

School

Your teacher is answering your question about the homework. The student behind you whispers that you're stupid.

Students are choosing sides for basketball. When you're chosen, they say you're a klutz.

On the way home some kids start calling you names: "Hey Fatso, Tubbo, Four-Eyes, Tinsel Teeth."

You're going to your special class. Some students tease you about being in the slow class.

Home Note

Client Name _____ Date _____

TODAY'S OBJECTIVE: Handle name-calling and teasing (take a deep breath to get calm; keep a pleasant face; look away or walk away if you can; say nice things to yourself by thinking, I am calm; I can ignore). When you handle name-calling and teasing you will feel better about yourself; people will tease you less; you won't get in arguments or fights.

TARGET BEHAVIORS: In addition to handling name-calling and teasing, the following individual skills were practiced.

	Score	Scale
A. _____ ____	1 = completely satisfied
B. _____ ____	2 = satisfied
C. _____ ____	3 = slightly satisfied
	4 = neither satisfied nor dissatisfied
D. _____ ____	5 = slightly dissatisfied
	6 = dissatisfied
E. _____ ____	7 = completely dissatisfied

The best thing done today: _____

_____

✂ —

PLEASE COMPLETE THIS SECTION AND RETURN

Client Name _____

SKILL 18: Handle name-calling and teasing

Did the participant use today's skill at least once this week?

	Yes	No
1. Take a deep breath to get calm.	____	____
2. Keep a pleasant face.	____	____
3. Look away or walk away if you can.	____	____
4. Say nice things to yourself by thinking, I am calm; I can ignore.	____	____

TARGET BEHAVIORS: Use the 1–7 scale to rate the target behaviors listed above.

COMMENTS:

A. ____

B. ____

C. ____

D. ____

E. ____

Signature _____ Date _____

SKILL 18: HANDLE NAME-CALLING AND TEASING   **Homework**

Client Name _____ Date _____

1. If someone at home or work teases you for being too slow, what can you do?

   _____

   _____

   _____

   _____

   _____

2. Say two nice things about yourself.

   a. _____

   b. _____

3. What can you do if someone doesn't stop teasing you?

   _____

   _____

   _____

   _____

   _____

Skill 19: Share

> Follow the instructions provided in Session Outline 2 for conducting • Conversation Time and Homework Completion and • Relaxation Training. Then go on to the • Skill Lesson.

SKILL LESSON

Introduce skill and list components.

Instructor 1: *(Ask participants to form a circle.)* Today we are going to talk about how to share. To share, you:

- Use a pleasant face and voice.

- Divide something so others can have some, too.

- Or take turns.

Role-play appropriate example.

Instructor 1: This is the right way to share. There's only one cookie left, and my roommate comes in.

Instructor 2: Hi, what are you doing?

Instructor 1: I'm having a snack. Would you like half of this cookie?

Ask participants for skill components.

Instructor 1: How did you know that was the right way to share? *(Participants respond or are prompted.)*

Role-play inappropriate example.

Instructor 1: This is the wrong way to share. There's only one cookie left, and my roommate comes in.

Instructor 2: Hi, what are you doing?

Instructor 1: I'm having a snack. It's the last cookie. (Eats it.)

Ask participants for skill components.

Instructor 1: What should have happened to make that the right way to share? *(Participants respond or are prompted.)*

Ask participants to role-play.

Instructor 1: Now it's your turn to role-play. I am going to call on someone who has been working really hard in the group today by (name specific on-task behaviors). _____ has been (name appropriate behaviors) and looks ready to be the first one to role-play. _____, this is your role-play.

(Describe the role-play you have previously selected for this participant from the role-play chart following this session outline. Have each participant role-play the skill correctly at least once, using a previously selected situation.)

Ask participants to give positive feedback.

Instructor 1 or 2: Good role-playing. Who can tell _____ what he/she did right to share in the role-play? *(Call on a participant who is volunteering and paying attention.)*

Ask participants for rationales for using skill.

Instructor 1: Why do you think it is important to share? *(Participants respond or are prompted.)*

Possible responses:

- Others will want to share with you.

- You will make more friends.

- You will make others feel good.

- People will like you.

Lead participants through reality check.

Instructor 1: Sometimes you try really hard to share, and this might happen. There's only one cookie left, and my roommate comes in.

Instructor 2: Hi, what are you doing?

Instructor 1: I'm having a snack. Would you like half of this cookie?

Instructor 2: No, I want all of it. I'm really hungry, and I made those cookies! (Grabs cookie.)

Instructor 1: You just did everything right to share. What should you do if this happens to you? *(Participants respond or are prompted.)*

Possible responses:

- Take a deep breath to get calm.

- Show a good attitude.

- Ask the person nicely to share with you.

- Ignore the person and find something else to do.

Follow the instructions provided in Session Outline 2 for conducting • Refreshment Time • Activity • Home Notes and • New Homework.

Suggested activities for Session 19: Marble Game, Greeting Game—see Appendix B.

Role-Plays

Home

You're eating out with your family, and there's only one piece of pizza left.

You're watching music videos on TV. Your roommate comes in and says her favorite program is on and she'd like to watch it.

You and another resident in the group home get to the bathroom at the same time to brush your teeth before you go to work.

Your supervisor found your apartment a mess. You and your roommate have 1 hour to clean it up.

Community

You are doing laundry in the laundry room at your apartment, and you and your roommate need a dryer at the same time.

You go bowling with a friend, and you both want to use the same ball.

You and two friends are taking the bus to the mall, and there is only room for two to sit down. It's a long ride.

At Special Olympics ski practice there are not enough skis for everyone to ski at the same time.

Work

You're sitting at a table alone at lunch. Two workers come in and don't know where to sit.

You're at work eating lunch, and you have two chocolate chip cookies. A coworker comes up and says, "Those are my favorite."

Two of you would like to take your break now, but only one of you can go at a time.

The supervisor says three of you can leave when the floor is swept and mopped. There is only one mop and one broom.

School

You want to talk to your teacher after class, but he's talking to two other students. You heard him say he had to leave in 10 minutes.

One of your friends wants to play soccer, and another wants to play kickball. You are in charge of the ball.

You want to go to the listening center. Only one person can use it at a time; two of you get there at the same time.

Your friend forgot his pencil today. You have an extra one.

Home Note

Client Name _____ Date _____

TODAY'S OBJECTIVE: Share (use a pleasant face and voice; divide something so others can have some, too; or take turns). When you share others will want to share with you; you will make more friends; you will make others feel good; people will like you.

TARGET BEHAVIORS: In addition to sharing, the following individual skills were practiced.

	Score	**Scale**
A. _____ ____		1 = completely satisfied
B. _____ ____		2 = satisfied
		3 = slightly satisfied
C. _____ ____		4 = neither satisfied nor dissatisfied
D. _____ ____		5 = slightly dissatisfied
		6 = dissatisfied
E. _____ ____		7 = completely dissatisfied

The best thing done today: _____

_____

✂ —

PLEASE COMPLETE THIS SECTION AND RETURN

Client Name _____

SKILL 19: Share

Did the participant use today's skill at least once this week?

	Yes	No
1. Use a pleasant face and voice.	____	____
2. Divide something so others can have some, too.	____	____
3. Or take turns.	____	____

TARGET BEHAVIORS: Use the 1–7 scale to rate the target behaviors listed above.

COMMENTS:

A. ____

B. ____

C. ____

D. ____

E. ____

Signature _____ Date _____

Homework

Client Name _____ Date _____

1. Write down two times you shared at home, at work, or elsewhere this week.

   Time 1:

   a. With whom did you share? _____

   b. How did you share? _____

   _____

   Time 2:

   a. With whom did you share? _____

   b. How did you share? _____

   _____

2. Give three reasons why it is good to share with others.

   a. _____

   b. _____

   c. _____

3. Tell about a time someone shared with you and how it made you feel.

   a. How did the other person share? _____

   _____

   b. How did you feel? _____

   _____

Skill 20: Compromise

> Follow the instructions provided in Session Outline 2 for
> conducting • Conversation Time and Homework Completion
> and • Relaxation Training. Then go on to the • Skill Lesson.

SKILL LESSON

Introduce skill and list components.

Instructor 1: *(Ask participants to form a circle.)* Today we are
going to talk about how to compromise. To
compromise, you:

- Use a pleasant face and voice.
- Think of a way both people can get something
  they want.
- Suggest it.

Role-play appropriate example.

Instructor 1: This is the right way to compromise. My boyfriend/
girlfriend comes over to take me on a date.

Instructor 2: I'd like my friend Jim to come with us to dinner and
the movie.

Instructor 1: (Uses pleasant face and voice.) Well, I wanted to be
alone with you.

Instructor 2: I haven't seen him in a long time.

Instructor 1: Well, how about if you and I go out to eat together,
and Jim can meet us for the movie?

Instructor 2: OK.

Ask participants for skill components.

Instructor 1: How did you know that was the right way to compromise? *(Participants respond or are prompted.)*

Role-play inappropriate example.

Instructor 1: This is the wrong way to compromise. My boyfriend/
girlfriend comes over to take me on a date.

Instructor 2: I'd like my friend Jim to come with us to dinner and the movie.

Instructor 1: Well, I wanted to be alone with you.

Instructor 2: I haven't seen him in a long time.

Instructor 1: I don't like that idea. I guess we can't go out tonight.

Ask participants for skill components.

Instructor 1: What should have happened to make that the right way to compromise? *(Participants respond or are prompted.)*

Ask participants to role-play.

Instructor 1: Now it's your turn to role-play. I am going to call on someone who has been working really hard in the group today by (name specific on-task behaviors). _____ has been (name appropriate behaviors) and looks ready to be the first one to role-play. _____, this is your role-play.

(Describe the role-play you have previously selected for this participant from the role-play chart following this session outline. Have each participant role-play the skill correctly at least once, using a previously selected situation.)

Ask participants to give positive feedback.

• Instructor 1 or 2: Good role-playing. Who can tell _____ what he/she did right to compromise in the role-play? *(Call on a participant who is volunteering and paying attention.)*

Ask participants for rationales for using skill.

Instructor 1: Why do you think it is important to compromise? *(Participants respond or are prompted.)*

Possible responses:

- People will try to compromise with you.

- People will feel good about doing things with you.

- Each person gets a little of what he or she wants.

Lead participants through reality check.

Instructor 1: Sometimes you try really hard to compromise, and this might happen. My boyfriend/girlfriend comes over to take me on a date.

Instructor 2: I'd like my friend Jim to come with us to dinner and the movie.

Instructor 1: (Uses pleasant face and voice.) Well, I wanted to be alone with you.

174

Instructor 2: I haven't seen him in a long time.

Instructor 1: Well, how about if you and I go out to eat together, and Jim can meet us for the movie?

Instructor 2: Well, I'm sorry, but either Jim comes with us or I guess we can't go out tonight.

Instructor 1: You just did everything right to compromise. What should you do if this happens to you? *(Participants respond or are prompted.)*

Possible responses:

- Take a deep breath to get calm.

- Keep a good attitude.

- Try to compromise again later.

Follow the instructions provided in Session Outline 2 for conducting • Refreshment Time • Activity • Home Notes and • New Homework.

Suggested activities for Session 20: Board Games, Marble Game, Greeting Game—see Appendix B.

Role-Plays

Home

You are really hungry. Dinner will be late because the meal planners didn't plan well. What can you do or say?

The weekend activities are being planned at a family meeting. You want to go somewhere; everyone else wants to stay home.

Your parents volunteered you to help your aunt clean her garage on Saturday. You have plans with your friends.

You haven't had a roommate for nearly a month. Today a new person is moving in. How will you both use the closet?

Community

You and two friends are ordering a pizza. What toppings will you have on it?

You are shopping for dinner with your roommate. You want spaghetti; your roommate wants macaroni and cheese.

Your girlfriend/boyfriend wants to go out dancing. You want a quiet evening at home.

You and a friend are going home on the bus. You are both tired of standing; one seat is empty.

Work

You need help lifting some boxes. A coworker needs help loading the truck.

Some coworkers are sending out for sandwiches for lunch. You wanted to go to the deli.

Your supervisor wants you to teach a new person your job. You wanted to ask for a day off, but you are now afraid you will lose your job if you ask.

You need to leave in 10 minutes for a dental appointment. Your boss wants the floor swept before you go.

School

Your teacher asks for volunteers to show the new student around school. Three of you raise your hands at the same time.

In living skills class, four of you must plan a meal to cook. Everyone wants to make dessert.

You and your friends are trying to decide what game to play.

A friend asks to have lunch with you. You already promised another friend you'd eat with her.

Home Note

Client Name _____ Date _____

TODAY'S OBJECTIVE: Compromise (use a pleasant face and voice; think of a way both people can get something they want; suggest it). When you compromise people will try to compromise with you; people will feel good about doing things with you; each person gets a little of what he or she wants.

TARGET BEHAVIORS: In addition to compromising, the following individual skills were practiced.

	Score	Scale
A. _____ ____		1 = completely satisfied
B. _____ ____		2 = satisfied
		3 = slightly satisfied
C. _____ ____		4 = neither satisfied nor dissatisfied
D. _____ ____		5 = slightly dissatisfied
		6 = dissatisfied
E. _____ ____		7 = completely dissatisfied

The best thing done today: _____

_____

✂ —

PLEASE COMPLETE THIS SECTION AND RETURN

Client Name _____

SKILL 20: Compromise

Did the participant use today's skill at least once this week?

	Yes	No
1. Use a pleasant face and voice.	____	____
2. Think of a way both people can get something they want.	____	____
3. Suggest it.	____	____

TARGET BEHAVIORS: Use the 1–7 scale to rate the target behaviors listed above.

COMMENTS:

A. ____

B. ____

C. ____

D. ____

E. ____

Signature _____ Date _____

Homework

Client Name _____ Date _____

1. Write down two times you compromised with someone so you both got something you wanted.

   Time 1:

   a. What was the problem? _____

   _____

   b. What compromise did you come up with? _____

   _____

   Time 2:

   a. What was the problem? _____

   _____

   b. What compromise did you come up with? _____

   _____

2. Give two reasons why it is good to compromise.

   a. _____

   b. _____

3. What are three things you could do if you tried to compromise but the other person would not?

   a. _____

   b. _____

   c. _____

Skill 21: Ask for Clear Directions

> Follow the instructions provided in Session Outline 2 for conducting • Conversation Time and Homework Completion and • Relaxation Training. Then go on to the • Skill Lesson.

SKILL LESSON

Introduce skill and list components.

Instructor 1: *(Ask participants to form a circle.)* Today we are going to talk about how to ask for clear directions. To ask for clear directions, you:

- Use a pleasant face and voice.

- Look at the person.

- Ask for more information or say, "I don't understand."

- Listen to the person.

- Repeat the directions to the person to show you understand.

Role-play appropriate example.

Instructor 1: This is the right way to ask for clear directions. I'm at work, and my supervisor gives me some directions.

Instructor 2: (Instructor 1), I'd like you to clean up the mess we left.

Instructor 1: (Uses pleasant face and voice, looks at supervisor.) OK . . . What do I do?

Instructor 2: I want you to sweep the floor and stack the boxes in the corner.

Instructor 1: OK. You want me to clean the floor and put the boxes over there.

Instructor 2: Yes, that's right.

Ask participants for skill components.

Instructor 1: How did you know that was the right way to ask for clear directions? *(Participants respond or are prompted.)*

Role-play inappropriate example.

Instructor 1: This is the wrong way to ask for clear directions. I'm at work, and my supervisor gives me some directions.

Instructor 2: (Instructor 1), I'd like you to clean up the mess we left.

Instructor 1: OK. I'll do it right away.

Ask participants for skill components.

Instructor 1: What should have happened to make that the right way to ask for clear directions? *(Participants respond or are prompted.)*

Ask participants to role-play.

Instructor 1: Now it's your turn to role-play. I am going to call on someone who has been working really hard in the group today by (name specific on-task behaviors). _____ has been (name appropriate behaviors) and looks ready to be the first one to role-play. _____, this is your role-play.

(Describe the role-play you have previously selected for this participant from the role-play chart following this session outline. Have each participant role-play the skill correctly at least once, using a previously selected situation.)

Ask participants to give positive feedback.

Instructor 1 or 2: Good role-playing. Who can tell _____ what he/she did right to ask for clear directions in the role-play? *(Call on a participant who is volunteering and paying attention.)*

Ask participants for rationales for using skill.

Instructor 1: Why do you think it is important to ask for clear directions? *(Participants respond or are prompted.)*

Possible responses:

- You won't make mistakes as often.

- You will know exactly what to do.

- People will get along better.

Lead participants through reality check.

Instructor 1: Sometimes you try really hard to ask for clear directions, and this might happen. I'm at work, and my supervisor gives me some directions.

Instructor 2: (Instructor 1), I'd like you to clean up the mess we left.

Instructor 1: (Uses pleasant face and voice, looks at supervisor.) OK . . . What do I do?

Instructor 2: Now (Instructor 1), you know what to do. Just go and do it and stop wasting my time!

Instructor 1: You just did everything right to ask for clear directions. What should you do if this happens to you? *(Participants respond or are prompted.)*

Possible responses:

- Take a deep breath to get calm.

- Keep a good attitude.

- Do the best job you can anyway.

- Try again later to ask for clear directions.

Follow the instructions provided in Session Outline 2 for conducting • Refreshment Time • Activity • Home Notes and • New Homework.

Suggested activities for Session 21: Directed Drawing, Treasure Hunt—see Appendix B.

Role-Plays

Home

Your mom can show you how to hook up your stereo if you ask her.

Your home manager announces the project for the day is spring cleaning. Your assignment is the family room.

The supervisor says no one is to leave the apartment until it is absolutely clean.

It's your day to do laundry, but you forgot how to operate the washer.

Community

You need to go to the post office for stamps, but you forgot how to get there.

Your church is having a work day to plant flowers. John is the man in charge. You came to help.

You are having dinner out with your friend at a new restaurant, and you have to go to the rest room.

You are going to the mall, and you think you might be on the wrong bus.

Work

Your supervisor wants you to get some papers copied for her.

When you get to work, your work group is rearranging the lunch room.

Your boss says you put the wrong nuts on the bolts, so you need to do them again right.

A coworker comes to you, saying, "The supervisor says get some people and get everything off the floor."

School

Your teacher wants you to take a message.

A classmate is fixing the calendar for the new month. The teacher said you could help.

Some students are playing a new soccer game. You want to learn how to play it with them.

The teacher said you could clean the chalkboard. You start, and he says, "No, no. You're making too big of a mess."

Home Note

Client Name _____ Date _____

TODAY'S OBJECTIVE: Ask for clear directions (use a pleasant face and voice; look at the person; ask for more information or say, "I don't understand"; listen to the person; repeat the directions to the person to show you understand). When you ask for clear directions you won't make mistakes as often; you will know exactly what to do; people will get along better.

TARGET BEHAVIORS: In addition to asking for clear directions, the following individual skills were practiced.

	Score	**Scale**
A. _____ ____		1 = completely satisfied
B. _____ ____		2 = satisfied
C. _____ ____		3 = slightly satisfied
D. _____ ____		4 = neither satisfied nor dissatisfied
E. _____ ____		5 = slightly dissatisfied
		6 = dissatisfied
		7 = completely dissatisfied

The best thing done today: _____

_____

✂ —

PLEASE COMPLETE THIS SECTION AND RETURN

Client Name _____

SKILL 21: Ask for clear directions

Did the participant use today's skill at least once this week?

	Yes	No
1. Use a pleasant face and voice.	____	____
2. Look at the person.	____	____
3. Ask for more information or say, "I don't understand."	____	____
4. Listen to the person.	____	____
5. Repeat the directions to the person to show you understand.	____	____

TARGET BEHAVIORS: Use the 1–7 scale to rate the target behaviors listed above.

COMMENTS:

A. ____
B. ____
C. ____
D. ____
E. ____

Signature _____ Date _____

Homework

Client Name _____ Date _____

1. Write down two directions someone gave you that you did not understand. Tell what you said and did to ask for clear directions and what the other person said and did.

   Direction 1:

   a. What did you say and do? _____

   _____

   b. What did the other person say and do? _____

   _____

   Direction 2:

   a. What did you say and do?_____

   _____

   b. What did the other person say and do?_____

   _____

2. When you don't understand, why is it important to ask for clear directions?

   _____

   _____

   _____

3. When you are giving directions, why should you try to make them as clear as possible?

   _____

   _____

   _____

4. What happens when you don't understand the directions, and you don't ask for clear directions?

   _____

   _____

   _____

APPENDIXES

Supplemental Training Materials

APPENDIX A

Relaxation Training Scripts

SCRIPT 1: TENSING AND RELAXING

We are going to practice relaxing together. Relaxing is learning to be calm in every part of your body. Relaxing makes your body feel calm and soft from your toes to the top of your head. Most of the day we are walking around or sitting in a chair. Your body works hard all day to hold you up. When you get tired at night, you go to sleep. Sleep gives your body rest, peace, and quiet. Your body relaxes when you sleep. We will relax without falling asleep. You can relax and stay awake. To learn to relax, we will start by (lying on the floor/sitting in a chair). Find a place where you have room to stretch out. *(Use Ignore-Attend-Praise to encourage participants to get into a relaxed position.)*

Some people like to close their eyes to relax. Others like to keep their eyes partly open. Let your eyes relax and do what feels comfortable to you. Let your feet (flop/rest flat on the floor). Place your hands comfortably (at your sides/on your lap). Your body is in a straight line. Feel your body (lying on the floor/sitting in the chair). Feel how the (floor/chair) touches the different parts of your body, your legs, buttocks, back, shoulders, arms. Feel your whole body being held up by the (floor/chair). Your body feels soft and warm and relaxed.

Let your breath go quietly in and out of your body. Think about how your body feels (on the floor/in the chair). Notice the body parts I am going to talk about and let them get softer and relaxed.

Tensing and then relaxing your muscles will help you feel even more relaxed. First, think about your right hand. Make a tight fist with your hand, as if you are squeezing something in your hand as hard as you can. Show me your fist. Notice how your fist feels. It may feel uncomfortable, and you can feel your muscles being tight and stretched. Now relax your hand by letting the muscles go soft and loose. Notice how your hand feels when it is relaxed. It feels warm and soft, with the muscles in your hand and fingers being relaxed and loose. Now we are going to practice tensing and relaxing different parts of our bodies, noticing the difference between being tight and tense, and being soft and relaxed.

Let's start with your feet. Tense your feet by pushing your toes against the top of your shoes. Feel how hard your foot muscles feel. Now relax by letting your feet go loose and soft. Feel the warm, tingly feeling in your feet. This is how it feels when your muscles relax.

Next think about your lower legs, where your calf muscles are. Tense your calf muscles by pushing your heels down. Feel the backs of your legs become hard and stretched. Now relax by letting your heels move up. Your calf muscles feel calm and soft and relaxed. *(Pause.)*

Now we will work on your thigh muscles in your upper legs, the muscles between your knees and your hips. Tighten your upper leg muscles as tight as you can while you keep the rest of your body relaxed. Feel how tight they are. Now let your legs go limp, and as you do, notice how relaxed they are becoming.

Now think about your stomach and chest. Tense the muscles here by holding in your stomach and holding your breath at the same time. Feel how tight your stomach muscles feel. Now relax by letting your breath out and your stomach go soft. It feels better to let your muscles relax.

Next think about your shoulders. Tense your shoulder muscles by pulling your shoulders up toward your ears. Keep your shoulders tensed, feeling how tight they feel. Now relax, letting your shoulders go down and your neck muscles go soft and relaxed. That feels better, doesn't it?

Now we are going to tense our arms. Tense your arm muscles by bending your arms and tightening up the muscles. Clench your fists, too, so all the muscles of both arms feel hard. Now relax by letting your arms and hands become soft and floppy. Feel the warm, soft, tingly feeling in your arms and hands. *(Pause.)*

Think about your head and face. Tense your head and face muscles by making a tight face, pressing your lips together, and scrunching up your forehead. Feel the tension making the muscles feel tight and hard. Relax, letting your face go soft, and feel how the tension leaves your face and head. There is less tension in your body now than when we started. Your whole body feels soft, calm, and relaxed.

Now, tense all your muscles. Tense your legs, your stomach, your arms, your hands, and your face. Your whole body feels hard and stretched tight, like a rubber band that is stretched until it almost breaks. Now relax. Feel your whole body become soft and warm and relaxed, like it's sinking into the (floor/chair).

It helps to practice tensing and relaxing every day. Just before you go to sleep, you can practice tensing and relaxing parts of your body while you lie on your bed. You can also practice tensing and relaxing whenever you feel upset or have a problem to solve. It can help you to stop and think before you do something.

In a few seconds, I will tell you to open your eyes and come back to the group. You will feel relaxed and ready for our lesson. *(Pause.)* Now slowly open your eyes.

SCRIPT 2: LEARNING TO BREATHE

Now we are going to practice relaxation. To be ready to relax, you need to get into a relaxing position by (lying on the floor/sitting in a chair), with your body in a straight line and feet (flopped/flat on the floor). Put your hands on your stomach or by your side. Good. *(Use Ignore-Attend-Praise to encourage participants to get into a relaxed position.)*

Think about how your muscles feel; if some of them feel tight, tense them and then relax them, making them soft and comfortable. Today we are going to relax by taking big, slow breaths.

Think about your breathing. The air gently goes in and out of your body. When you breathe in, the air goes into your lungs. The air going in makes your chest bigger. When you breathe really big and slow, your stomach gets bigger, too. When you breathe out, your stomach and chest will get smaller again. This big and slow breathing is called *stomach breathing.* It helps your whole body relax when you breathe so big that your stomach moves.

Remember that you learned to relax your muscles by tightening and relaxing parts of your body. You did that by thinking with your mind. You relaxed your muscles by thinking about them one at a time. Remember how calm and relaxed your whole body felt. Another way to relax is to breathe big and slow. Today we will practice big, slow breathing.

Relax your eyes by closing them. Place your hands on your stomach to feel your breath going in and out of your body. Feel your body get soft and be held up by the (floor/chair). Feel your body relaxing. Breathe in. Breathe out.

With your hands on your stomach, you will feel your stomach get bigger when you breathe in. I will say, "Breathe in, 1 . . . 2," and you will breathe in a big, slow breath. Then I will say, "Breathe out, 1 . . . 2." You will let your breath out slowly. Each time you practice breathing and relaxing, it will be easier to do. You will feel more and more relaxed. You will feel good about learning to do a new thing. Let's practice big, slow breathing again. I will give directions, and you will breathe and relax.

Breathe in, 1 . . . 2 *(pause)*. Breathe out, 1 . . . 2. Feel your stomach get big as the air goes in and small as the air goes out. Breathe in, 1 . . . 2 *(pause)*. Breathe out, 1 . . . 2. Good. Feel your body getting more relaxed. Breathe in, 1 . . . 2 *(pause)*. Breathe out, 1 . . . 2. Let all your breath out. Breathe in, 1 . . . 2 *(pause)*. Breathe out, 1 . . . 2. Each time you breathe out, you feel more and more relaxed. I can see that you all (or name specific individuals) are relaxing the right way by keeping your eyes closed, resting your hands on your stomachs, and letting your feet relax. Keep breathing big and slow, and I will talk about another thing to do while you are breathing.

Picture the air coming in and out of your body, and as you breathe out, say out loud, "I am calm." Breathe in slowly, and then as you breathe out say softly, "I am calm." Let's practice breathing with saying, "I am calm." I will say, "Breathe in, 1 . . . 2 *(pause)*. Breathe out," and we will say, "I am calm" together. Here we go.

Breathe in, 1 . . . 2 *(pause)*. Breathe out, saying, "I am calm." Breathe in, making your stomach big. Breathe out, saying, "I am calm." Good. Breathe in, 1 . . . 2 *(pause)*. Breathe out, "I am calm." Breathe in, 1 . . . 2 *(pause)*. Breathe out, "I am calm." I can hear everyone (or name individuals following directions) saying, "I am calm." Breathe in, 1 . . . 2 *(pause)*. Breathe out, "I am calm." One more time. Breathe in, 1 . . . 2. Breathe out, "I am calm." Now relax and breathe as you usually do, quietly. Your body feels relaxed and soft.

What a good job everyone did, practicing stomach breathing with big, slow breaths. We will practice relaxing each time we meet. You can practice at home and at work, too. The more you practice breathing and relaxing, the easier it will be. Then you can breathe and relax whenever you need to get calm and think better.

To finish relaxing, open your eyes and slowly sit up. I will know you are ready for the lesson when you are sitting up and looking at me. Thank you for listening and relaxing.

SCRIPT 3: GUIDED IMAGERY

You have learned some different ways to relax. You learned to make your muscles relax. You learned to take big, slow breaths and say, "I am calm."

Sometimes, when you do something new like a class or job, or when you meet a new person, you might feel uncomfortable or nervous. Relaxing can make you feel better. Sometimes you may have a problem. You might feel frustrated or angry. Relaxing can help you feel better so you can think. When you can think, you can solve problems. It is hard to think when you feel tense. You can make your mind work for you by relaxing. To be ready to relax, get into a relaxing position by (lying on the floor/sitting in a chair), with your body in a straight line and feet (flopped/flat on the floor). *(Use Ignore-Attend-Praise to encourage participants to get into a relaxed position.)*

Put your hands on your stomach or by your side. Good. Think about how your muscles feel; if some of them feel tight, tense them and then relax them, making them soft and comfortable. Relax your eyes by closing them. Feel your body get soft and be held up by the (floor/chair). Feel your body relaxing. Breathe in. Breathe out.

First, we will practice breathing as we did before, only this time, instead of saying, "I am calm" out loud, think it to yourself. I will say, "Breathe in, 1 . . . 2." Then I will say, "Breathe out and think, I am calm." Let's try it.

Breathe in, 1 . . . 2 *(pause)*. Breathe out and think, I am calm. Good. Breathe in, 1 . . . 2 *(pause)*. Breathe out and think, I am calm. Feel the (floor/chair) holding your body. Breathe in, 1 . . . 2 *(pause)*. Breathe out . . . I am calm. Feel your stomach move as you breathe. Breathe in, 1 . . . 2 *(pause)*. Breathe out . . . I am calm. Think to yourself as you relax. Breathe in, 1 . . . 2 *(pause)*. Breathe out, I am calm. Good. Now you are more relaxed.

Breathing and thinking, I am calm helps you feel calm and relaxed. You have learned how to make your body relaxed by tensing muscles and then relaxing them, taking big, slow breaths, and thinking, I am calm. You can do these things whenever and wherever you feel tense or worried or confused. You can make your body and your mind work for you to help you feel better.

Now we are going to practice another way to make your mind work for you. To make your mind work for you, you will breathe big and slow while I tell a story. As you listen to the story, make pictures about the story in your mind. It will be like a movie in your head. Close your eyes while I tell the story, and just listen to my words.

The story is about all of us going for a ride in a hot air balloon. First, we have to breathe big and slow to fill the hot air balloon. It is lying flat on the ground. Breathe in, 1 . . . 2. Breathe out, 1 . . . 2. Think of the sound of the air. Breathe in, 1 . . . 2. Breathe out, 1 . . . 2. It is almost full. Breathe in, 1 . . . 2. Breathe out, 1 . . . 2. The balloon is full of air and ready to go. Keep breathing in and out slowly. In your mind, we all get into the big basket under the balloon and wave good-bye to our friends on the ground. Going up in the air is so gentle, like going up in an elevator very slowly. We look around and see blue sky and the ground below us. There are the buildings we live in way below us. There are trees and grass. There is the workshop (name and describe locales participants are familiar with). Breathe in, 1 . . . 2. Breathe out, 1 . . . 2. It's so calm and quiet up here. Keep breathing big and slow as the balloon goes over our community. Now our balloon is floating toward (name location of the group), where people we know are outside waving to us. We are floating down to them, feeling calm and relaxed. They are all smiling, and so are we. Breathe in . . . breathe out. The balloon is going down. Our friends are waiting for us. The basket touches on the ground, and we climb out to greet our friends. Breathe in . . . breathe out. The balloon ride is finished, and our minds are slowly bringing us back to this room, feeling relaxed and calm.

Our minds took us on a wonderful trip. You feel happy, and your body feels calm and relaxed. We will practice this again so you can feel calm and relaxed whenever you want to. When you feel calm and relaxed, you will feel better and be able to solve problems.

Now think about this room, the chairs, where you are (on the floor/sitting), who is in the room with you. When you can picture the room, open your eyes, still breathing big and slow. When you are ready, sit up and form a circle. Then we will be ready for today's lesson.

SCRIPT 4: IMAGERY FOR INDIVIDUAL SKILLS

> This script is written for Skill 4, following directions. Adapt it to fit other skills as needed.

Today we are going to relax again. We will be remembering the difference between being relaxed and tense, and using deep breathing to help us become very relaxed. To be ready to relax, get into a relaxing position by (lying on the floor/sitting in a chair), with your body in a straight line and feet (flopped/flat on the floor). *(Use Ignore-Attend-Praise to encourage participants to get into a relaxed position.)*

First, think about your right hand. Make a tight fist with your hand, as if you are squeezing something in your hand as hard as you can. Show me your fist. Notice how your fist feels. It may feel uncomfortable, and you can feel your muscles being tight and stretched. Now relax your hand by letting the muscles go soft and loose. Notice how your hand feels when it is relaxed. It feels warm and soft, with the muscles in your hand and fingers being relaxed and loose. Now we are going to tense and relax your entire body. Make your whole body stiff like a board; push it down against the (floor/chair). Try to make a dent in the (floor/chair). *(Pause.)* Now relax. Feel the tightness drain out of your body. Feel the warm, soft, tingly feeling of your muscles being relaxed. It feels good.

Place your hands on your stomach to feel your breath going in and out of your body. Feel your body get soft and be held up by the (floor/chair). Feel your body relaxing. Breathe in. Breathe out.

With your hands on your stomach, you will feel your stomach get bigger when you breathe in. I will say, "Breathe in, 1 . . . 2," and you will breathe in a big, slow breath. Then I will say, "Breathe out, 1 . . . 2." You will let your breath out slowly.

Breathe in, 1 . . . 2 *(pause)*. Breathe out, 1 . . . 2. Feel your stomach get big as the air goes in and small as the air goes out. Breathe in, 1 . . . 2 *(pause)*. Breathe out, 1 . . . 2. Good. Feel your body getting more relaxed. Breathe in, 1 . . . 2 *(pause)*. Breathe out, 1 . . . 2. Let all your breath out. Breathe in, 1 . . . 2 *(pause)*. Breathe out, 1 . . . 2. Each time you breathe out, you feel more and more relaxed. I can see that you all (or name specific individuals) are relaxing the right way by keeping your eyes closed, resting your hands on your stomachs, and letting your feet relax.

Now that you are very relaxed, I want you to make believe with me. I want you to think of a time when you were upset or angry because someone asked you to do something you didn't want to do. Maybe it was late and your group home manager told you to turn off your radio. Maybe you were at work and someone told you that you had to finish a project before you could go on a break. (*Add relevant situations, if possible.*) Think of a time when someone gave you directions that you didn't like. How did you feel? Who was there? Were there any colors or sounds or smells you remember? Remember as many things as you can. Now, remember how you felt. Were you angry? Did you want to yell or cry? Did your stomach get upset? Did you feel your muscles being tense? Remember as many things as you can. *(Long pause.)*

Now we are going back to that time, and we are going to use our imaginations to change what happened. First, check your body to make sure you are very calm. *(Pause.)* Now imagine the person giving you directions that you don't like. This time you are very calm. Think of how you look. Think of how your body is when you are calm. The person is asking you to do something. You know you don't like it, but you decide to stay calm. You breathe deeply. You feel your muscles relax. You look at the person. You stay calm. You think about it. Maybe the group home manager has told you to turn off your radio. You know that by cooperating now you will have more privileges on the weekend. You remember how it feels to try to get up for work when you stay up too late. You say, "OK" in a calm voice. You do what the person asked. Maybe your supervisor told you to finish your project. You think about it. You remember that it is harder to remember what to do after your break. You take a deep breath, say, "OK," and finish the job. (*Follow up on specific situations added above.*) Take a few seconds to imagine yourself staying calm in your own situation. You look at the person. You stay calm. You think about it. You say, "OK."

Think about how you look staying calm and saying, "OK." Think about how your body is. Think about how your face looks. Notice how good you feel. Notice how strong you feel. Now, just notice your deep breathing and calm body for a few seconds. *(Pause.)* In a few seconds, I will tell you to open your eyes and come back in the group. You will feel relaxed and refreshed and ready for our lesson.

All right, now, begin to open your eyes. You feel very relaxed and refreshed. You feel very good. Open your eyes and we will go on to the lesson.

APPENDIX B

Suggested Activities

These activities accompany the 21 Skill Lessons presented in this book. For your convenience, the following list associates specific Skill Lessons with appropriate activities. In addition, the description of each activity includes a list of the skills it reinforces.

Our suggestions are by no means exhaustive, and we encourage your creativity. Modify or supplement the activities as you see fit. In modifying these activities or creating new ones, keep two goals in mind: First, an activity should suit the skills, interests, and capabilities of group members. Second, the activity should be an enjoyable way to practice a new skill.

Skill Lesson	Suggested Activities
1. Show a good attitude	Board Games (Activity 1) Musical Chairs (Activity 2) "May I" (Activity 3)
2. Have a calm body and voice	Board Games (Activity 1) Spoons (Activity 4)
3. Listen carefully	Simon Says (Activity 5) Telephone (Activity 6)
4. Follow directions	Simon Says (Activity 5) Directed Drawing (Activity 7) Marble Game (Activity 8)
5. Greet someone	Greeting Game (Activity 9)
6. Introduce yourself	Name Game (Activity 10)
7. Give positive feedback	Directed Drawing (Activity 7) Draw a Town (Activity 11)
8. Accept positive feedback	Draw a Town (Activity 11)
9. Interrupt the right way	Keeping Score (Activity 12)
10. Join in	Keeping Score (Activity 12) "Yes, and . . . " (Activity 13)
11. Ignore	Simon Says (Activity 5) Heroes and Villains (Activity 14) Teasing Game (Activity 15)

12. Accept no as an answer	"May I" (Activity 3) Marble Game (Activity 8)
13. Ask, don't tell	Board Games (Activity 1) Draw a Town (Activity 11)
14. Solve problems	Board Games (Activity 1) Problem Game (Activity 16)
15. Accept consequences	Board Games (Activity 1) Marble Game (Activity 8)
16. Take responsibility	Board Games (Activity 1) "May I" (Activity 3) Problem Game (Activity 16)
17. Say no to stay out of trouble	Heroes and Villains (Activity 14)
18. Handle name-calling and teasing	Heroes and Villains (Activity 14) Teasing Game (Activity 15)
19. Share	Marble Game (Activity 8) Greeting Game (Activity 9)
20. Compromise	Board Games (Activity 1) Marble Game (Activity 8) Greeting Game (Activity 9)
21. Ask for clear directions	Directed Drawing (Activity 7) Treasure Hunt (Activity 17)

ACTIVITY 1: BOARD GAMES

Skills   Show a good attitude (Skill 1)
                          Have a calm body and voice (Skill 2)
                          Ask, don't tell (Skill 13)
                          Solve problems (Skill 14)
                          Accept consequences (Skill 15)
                          Take responsibility (Skill 16)
                          Compromise (Skill 20)

Materials   Various board games

Process   Board games are good for practicing a variety of social skills. Select any games that are appropriate to the ages and abilities of participants. Allow a group of three or four to play each game. While they play, be ready to use the Teaching Strategies to teach appropriate interaction skills. For example, ask, don't tell may come up as one player attempts to "help" another play the game as he or she thinks it should be played.

ACTIVITY 2: MUSICAL CHAIRS

Skill   Show a good attitude (Skill 1)

Materials   Enough chairs for all participants but one
                          Music, either prerecorded or live

Process   This is the parlor and party game you probably played as a child. Have participants stand by the chairs, which have been arranged seats facing out in a circle in the middle of the room. Let the music begin. As the music plays, participants walk around outside the circle of chairs. Abruptly stop the music: All of the participants will scramble for a seat. The person without a seat must leave the game. The game continues with one person and one chair removed each round until only the winner is left in the game.

                          Because one person is always left without a seat, the game presents an opportunity to give Positive Feedback to those who show a good attitude.

ACTIVITY 3: "MAY I"

Skills   Show a good attitude (Skill 1)
                          Accept no as an answer (Skill 12)
                          Take responsibility (Skill 16)

Materials   A room with open space
                          Masking tape to mark finish line

Process   Use this script to introduce the game: "Today we are going to play a game called 'May I.' You may have played a game like this before, but I want you to listen carefully because the rules might be different. You will all start by standing in line along the wall on the other side of the room. After we start, you will have a turn when I call on you. When it is your turn, you may ask to take some steps toward the finish line. You may decide how many steps you want to ask for and what size steps to ask for. You can ask for tiny steps like this (show heel-to-toe steps), normal steps, or giant steps. Then I will say yes or no. If I say yes, you may take your steps. If I say no, then you won't be able to take the steps you asked for, but everyone else will. You will need to work especially hard to show a good attitude, accept no as an answer, and take responsibility. The first one to reach the finish line will win a prize."

Use the Teaching Strategies, especially Positive Feedback, to reinforce the appropriate skill(s). If a participant asks for an unreasonable number of steps (e.g., 20 giant steps), say no and let everyone else take the steps. Demonstrate the game with your teaching partner, if necessary. You may wish to give prizes after the game to those who did especially well at showing a good attitude, but do not announce this at the beginning. If players think they may get a prize anyway, the game will not be as effective at challenging their ability to accept no as an answer.

ACTIVITY 4: SPOONS

Skill

Have a calm body and voice (Skill 2)

Materials

One deck of playing cards per eight participants
One metal spoon for all but one participant

Process

Form groups of eight or fewer, with everyone seated on the floor or at a large table. The object of the game is to be the last person left after everyone else is eliminated.

Play begins with all of the spoons on the table or floor in front of the players. As in musical chairs, the number of spoons is one fewer than the number of players. As dealer, the instructor gives each player four cards. The object is to collect four of a kind—for example, four deuces or four kings. The dealer then passes cards one at a time around the circle, with each player deciding privately whether to pass the card on or keep it and pass a different one. Players keep only four cards at a time. A player who gets four of a kind may take a spoon. As soon as this happens, all other players must try to grab one, too. One player—and one spoon—is eliminated each round.

This game offers an enjoyable opportunity to use Positive Feedback and Ignore-Attend-Praise. Because spoon grabbing can be a frantic activity, watch for chances to reinforce participants for having a calm body and voice.

ACTIVITY 5: SIMON SAYS

Skill

Listen carefully (Skill 3)
Follow directions (Skill 4)
Ignore (Skill 11)

Materials

Small prizes

Process	Have participants form a circle and pick one participant to be "Simon." Tell participants to do whatever Simon says, as long as Simon begins the instruction with "Simon says . . ." Tell them to ignore other directions. If the participants are not familiar with this game, model instructions—for example, "Simon says raise your right hand. Simon says sit down. Simon says clap your hands three times. Touch your nose." Explain that you will keep score for correct imitation and give small prizes to those who have the highest scores at the end of the game.

Let the players take turns as Simon, praising volunteering and choosing those who have been listening, following directions, and ignoring distractions. You may model the skills by participating with the group.

ACTIVITY 6: TELEPHONE

Skill	Listen carefully (Skill 3)
Materials	Small prizes
Process	This activity is the familiar game of telephone, which tests how clearly a message can be transmitted through a series of people.

Have participants form a line or circle, seated in chairs or on the floor. Whisper a message in the ear of the first person. Each person relays this message to the next, with the last person saying what was heard.

Depending on the sophistication of the participants and their target behaviors, the message may be short or long, simple or complex. It might be related to the skill of listening carefully or to another skill already learned. For example, you could say, "To listen carefully, you must keep a quiet mouth."

Let a different person begin each round so that the last one to receive each message is also different. As the message is being whispered down the line, use Positive Feedback and Ignore-Attend-Praise to strengthen social skills, especially listening. To enhance the fun, you can give prizes to those who show good listening skills.

ACTIVITY 7: DIRECTED DRAWING

Skills	Follow directions (Skill 4) Give positive feedback (Skill 7) Ask for clear directions (Skill 21)
Materials	5 to 10 3- by 5-inch cards Drawing paper Pencils, markers, crayons, or other drawing materials
Process	Draw (or name) a simple item (e.g., house, tree, face, or shape) on each of the cards. Depending on the abilities of your group members, you may or may not want to show all of these before beginning the game. Depending on the verbal skills of the participants, one instructor may direct the game while the other uses the Teaching Strategies in incidental teaching.

Variation 1: Follow directions

Have group members work in pairs. One of each pair will be the "artist," and the other will give directions. The direction giver will pick a card, which the artist will not see. When ready, the direction giver will offer simple directions such as "Draw a circle in the middle of the page" or "Draw a line along the bottom of the page." The artist will follow the directions.

Variation 2: Give positive feedback

Play the game as described but have the individual providing the directions give positive feedback to the artist for drawing as instructed. (You may want to teach this skill incidentally whenever you play the game.)

Variation 3: Ask for clear directions

Play the game as described but prompt the artist to ask for more specifics and repeat them as directions are given.

ACTIVITY 8: MARBLE GAME

Skills

Follow directions (Skill 4)
Accept no as an answer (Skill 12)
Accept consequences (Skill 15)
Share (Skill 19)
Compromise (Skill 20)

Materials

A room with a lot of space, one empty wall, and an open floor
Marbles (one for each player)
Small prizes (candy, gum, erasers, etc.)
Paper cups with the words *give, get,* or *share* written on them (write the same word on three to five cups)

Process

Spread the prizes and labeled paper cups along the floor in front of the empty wall. Clear any furniture out of the way. Draw a chalk line (or stretch masking tape) parallel to and about 10 feet away from the prizes. Have the players sit behind the line. Give one marble to each player. Players take turns shooting and claiming any prizes their marbles hit. Use Positive Feedback to acknowledge those who show the necessary skill(s).

Rules

1. Players take turns in the order you establish.

2. Marbles leaving a player's hands out of turn will be confiscated, and the player will lose one turn.

3. A player may not shoot until the previous player has retrieved his or her marble and has returned behind the line.

4. If a player hits a cup, he or she does as instructed: Takes a prize (for *get*), returns a prize to the wall (for *give*), or shares a prize (for *share*).

5. You, the referee, will judge which prizes a marble has hit. If a player shoots before you are ready, that player will miss a turn.

ACTIVITY 9: GREETING GAME

Skills
Greet someone (Skill 5)
Share (Skill 19)
Compromise (Skill 20)

Materials
Crayons or markers, one fewer than the total number of participants in each group
A sheet of paper or newsprint for each participant

Process
Participants are each given a sheet of paper, and all but one is given a marker. Tell participants that they are to draw a picture of the group (or some other subject) and that they will need to borrow markers from one another in order to finish their pictures.

There are clear rules for borrowing markers: The person without a marker begins by choosing someone whose marker he or she wishes to borrow. The procedure is to practice greeting someone in the right way and then asking for the marker. If a correct greeting precedes the request, the person must give up the marker and get one from another player in the same way. If the borrower forgets to greet first, he or she does not get the marker and must try again with someone else.

The game is a chain exercise. That is, each borrower must approach and greet someone other than the person who just borrowed a marker from him or her. You may prompt to make sure that participants have an approximately equal number of turns. Be sure to give Positive Feedback for instances of sharing and compromising.

ACTIVITY 10: NAME GAME

Skill
Introduce yourself (Skill 6)

Materials
A set of cards naming movie or cartoon characters or animals with which participants are familiar (one card per player)
A pencil for each person and a piece of paper on which that person's name has been written
Small prizes

Process
Have each participant pick one card without revealing the name on it to anyone. Instruct participants to pretend to be the characters named on their cards. The object of the game is to learn the fictitious names of as many other players as possible in a set time (10 to 15 minutes). Participants should approach one another and introduce themselves, using their fictitious names, to as many other "characters" as they can. Instruct them to write down the fictitious names of the people they meet as they introduce themselves.

Give Positive Feedback to participants who are introducing themselves correctly. If some are not introducing themselves or are doing so incorrectly, use a Teaching Interaction or Ignore-Attend-Praise to help them practice the skill.

Rules

1. If a player makes a correct introduction by saying, "Hi," telling his or her name, and asking the other person's name, the other person must respond.

2. If a player fails to make a correct introduction, the other player does not have to respond. The first player must approach someone else.

3. When the time is up, everyone returns to the circle, and each player repeats the names of all the characters he or she has met.

4. A prize can be given to everyone who has learned the names of at least two or three characters.

ACTIVITY 11: DRAW A TOWN

Skills

Give positive feedback (Skill 7)
Accept positive feedback (Skill 8)
Ask, don't tell (Skill 13)

Materials

Multicolored paints, crayons, or markers for each group
A large sheet of butcher paper or newsprint for each group

Process

This activity is designed for four to six people. If you have eight or more, you may want to form more than one group.

Explain to group members that you want them to draw their neighborhood together. Each participant will have one color and one job to do. For example, the person with the black marker would draw the roads, while the one with the green marker would make grass and trees. The person with the brown marker would be in charge of making houses, and so on. Encourage group members to cooperate in deciding where to place the features of their neighborhood and to ask one another to add to the picture (e.g., ask the person with the red marker to draw a car on the road).

Point out and praise spontaneous occurrences of the skill you are working on. For example, watch for giving positive feedback: "Thank you for drawing a car on my road"; "Thanks for trading jobs with me"; "That's a good idea." Examples of accepting positive feedback and asking, not telling might respectively be "Thank you" and "Would you please put a road by my house?"

If a participant does not spontaneously use the desired skills, you can structure a practice situation. For example, if Jim does not use positive feedback, discreetly prompt the person working next to him to do something nice for Jim. If necessary, intervene with a Direct Prompt or a Teaching Interaction to help group members use the skills. You can also participate in the activity to model these skills.

ACTIVITY 12: KEEPING SCORE

Skills   Interrupt the right way (Skill 9)
                    Join in (Skill 10)

Materials   Chalkboard, flip chart, or other large area for keeping score

Process   Set up a score sheet that will be large enough for group members to see. Use the format illustrated, with participants' names listed along the left-hand side and four columns labeled at the top.

	Enter conversation	Wait for a pause	Excuse me or On topic	Interrupt
Joe				
Susan				
Greg				
Luke				
Erin				

During refreshment time or some other conversational activity, tell group members you will be keeping score on their conversations. Explain that they can earn 1 point for entering the conversation; 1 point for waiting for a pause; and 1 point for saying "Excuse me" (if teaching Skill 9) or for staying on the topic (if teaching Skill 10). However, they will lose 2 points for interrupting the wrong way (talking at the same time as another person). They must listen carefully to the other speakers so they don't interrupt the wrong way. Everyone must participate in the same conversation (i.e., not talk privately to a neighbor).

Total the points at the end of the game and give prizes for the best scores. Use your discretion; on some occasions, participants will accumulate many points, and other times only a few. By setting the criterion for winning, you can individualize the game for your group.

ACTIVITY 13: "YES, AND . . ."

Skill   Join in (Skill 10)

Materials   None

Process   Participants should be in groups of four to six. Explain that you want them to learn how to join in a conversation. Say that, by playing the "Yes, and . . ." game, they will learn how to become part of conversations with individuals or groups.

Have each small group pick a topic to discuss. You may need to assist by suggesting some neutral topic, such as the weather, clothes, and the like. When the topic has been chosen, a participant should speak on that topic for no more than a minute. When the first speaker finishes, the adjacent person joins in the conversation by saying, "Yes and . . ." This continues until all have spoken.

Some participants will only be able to complete a sentence; others will be able to expand significantly on the topic. Help each one feel successful by giving nonverbal reinforcement, timing your smiling and head nodding for the moment the person adds the first word to "Yes, and . . ."

When all participants have learned to join in successfully, you may wish to vary the game: Change the opening phrase to "Yes, but . . ." and thereafter to "Yes, if only . . ."

ACTIVITY 14: HEROES AND VILLAINS

Skills

Ignore (Skill 11)
Say no to stay out of trouble (Skill 17)
Handle name-calling and teasing (Skill 18)

Materials

For Variation 1:

A set of cards, each naming a well-known villain from a movie, cartoon strip, or TV series
Small prizes or edible treats

For Variation 2:

List of supervillains
List of superheroes
List of evil plots

Process

Variation 1: Ignore; handle name-calling and teasing

Have each participant pick one card. Then explain that each person will pretend to be the villain named on the chosen card. The group is seated in a circle. Each villain takes a turn sitting in the middle, first announcing the name on the card. The others name-call and tease the villain. Every villain who correctly and seriously ignores the teasing and handles the name-calling earns a prize. Give Positive Feedback, in addition to prizes, to those who successfully handle the name-calling.

Variation 2: Say no to stay out of trouble

Divide the participants into teams of two. Each team is assigned a supervillain, a superhero, and an evil plot. The group forms a circle, and teams take turns sitting in the middle. The villain of each team tries to talk the hero into helping with the evil plot; the hero practices saying no to stay out of trouble. The team members then trade roles.

Watch for instances of saying no appropriately, and respond with Positive Feedback. Use other Teaching Strategies as needed to help participants refine the skill.

ACTIVITY 15: TEASING GAME

Skills
Ignore (Skill 11)
Handle name-calling and teasing (Skill 18)

Materials
None

Process
Participants gather in one large circle. If you have 10 or more people, or if some have difficulty maintaining control, you may want to divide into smaller groups. Explain that you are going to practice dealing with teasing. Each participant takes a turn in the middle of the circle while the others try to tease him or her. Congratulate each participant on ignoring and handling name-calling and teasing.

ACTIVITY 16: PROBLEM GAME

Skills
Solve problems (Skill 14)
Take responsibility (Skill 16)

Materials

For Variation 1:

A list of problems, each of which implies several possible solutions
A large piece of paper and a marker
Small prizes

For Variation 2:

A list of problem situations in which something has happened and someone is in trouble as a result
Small prizes

Process

Variation 1: Solve problems

Divide the group into teams of two or three and have each team pick a leader. Then present a situational problem. You may want to use role-plays that were not used during the lesson, or you may choose specific problems that your group is facing. Some universal issues concern dating and sexuality, friendship and confidentiality, work and home, family versus friendships, values versus behavior (what we believe as opposed to what we do), and reconciling differences by negotiating.

Give each team the same problem. The team must discuss the problem and come up with three ideas for solving it. Then they choose the one they think is the best solution. Have each team leader present that solution to the whole group and tell why the team chose it. List the solutions on a large piece of paper and have the group vote on the best solution. Award a prize to the team whose solution wins. Repeat the exercise if time permits.

In addition to the main skill of solving problems, watch for chances to use Positive Feedback for cooperation, joining in, and following rules.

Variation 2: Take responsibility

Have participants form a circle; each participant takes a turn in the center. Present the participant with a problem. (You may use leftover role-plays from the lesson, if desired.) Have the participant tell the group what he or she would do in the situation. Give Positive Feedback and award prizes to participants whose solutions would let them take responsibility by being honest, not blaming others, and accepting consequences with a good attitude. Use other Teaching Strategies to help participants refine the skill.

ACTIVITY 17: TREASURE HUNT

Skill

Ask for clear directions (Skill 21)

Materials

Small pieces of paper for clues (2 per participant)
Small prizes

Process

Ahead of time, select hiding places in the room you will be using. You will need one hiding place per participant. For example:

- In the second drawer of the desk

- Under the pencil sharpener

- Behind a red chair

- Under a candy jar

Devise a clue that describes some characteristic of each hiding place. For example:

- In the second drawer of the desk *(middle)*

- Under the pencil sharpener *(point)*

- Behind a red chair *(red)*

- Under a candy jar *(sweet)*

Write each clue on two pieces of paper. Hide one of the pieces of paper in the corresponding hiding place (e.g., hide the paper that says *red* behind the red chair) and keep one to give to the player. Take notes as follows so you can remember who is looking for what and where it is hidden:

- In the second drawer of the desk *(middle)*: Sam

- Under the pencil sharpener *(point)*: Trish

- Behind a red chair *(red)*: Jay

- Under a candy jar *(sweet)*: Chris

Use the following script to introduce the game, demonstrating with your teaching partner if necessary: "Today we are going to have a treasure hunt. In a minute I will give each of you a clue that will help you find a matching ticket. When you have both matching tickets, you will get a prize. When I give you your clue, read it or ask me what it says. That will tell you something about the hiding place you are trying to find. Then you can ask me questions about the hiding place. You can ask things like 'Which side of the room is it on?' or 'What color is it?' When you think you have a good idea of where to look, ask me for permission to look. If your idea is close, then I will let you go look. If I say no, then you need to ask more questions to narrow it down."

Next give each clue to the proper person. After receiving the clues, participants may take turns asking for clear directions. Let participants ask as many questions as necessary to develop an idea about where to look. Require them to ask permission before looking for their clues. To prevent aimless and disruptive searching, ask them to be specific about where they want to look. Remember, the point of the game is to give them opportunities to ask for clear directions. When you are satisfied that a participant has asked enough questions and has a good idea of where to look, give permission to look for the clue. Continue the game until all have found their clues. When participants have found their clues, you may award them a small prize or privilege.

References

Christoff, K., & Kelly, J. (1983). Social skills. In J. L. Matson & S. E. Breuning (Eds.), *Assessing the mentally retarded.* New York: Grune & Stratton.

Conger, J. C., & Conger, A. J. (1982). Components of heterosocial competence. In J. P. Curran & P. M. Monti (Eds.), *Social skills training: A practical handbook for assessment and treatment.* New York: Guilford.

Curran, J. P. (1982). A procedure for the assessment of social skills: The simulated social interaction test. In J. P. Curran & P. M. Monti (Eds.), *Social skills training: A practical handbook for assessment and treatment.* New York: Guilford.

Miller, L. C. (1977). *Louisville Behavior Checklist.* Los Angeles: Western Psychological Services.

Strohmer, D. C., & Prout, H. T. (1989). *Strohmer-Prout Behavior Rating Scale.* Schenectady, NY: Genium.

About the Authors

Donald A. Jackson

Donald A. Jackson received his master's degree in psychology from Western Michigan University and his doctorate in 1973 from the University of Utah. He is Clinical Director and Psychologist for community programs at Northern Nevada Mental Retardation Services and Adjunct Professor in the Department of Psychology at the University of Nevada, Reno. He coauthored *Getting Along With Others: Teaching Social Effectiveness to Children* and has contributed numerous papers, presentations, and workshops on social skills training for children and for people with developmental disabilities.

Nancy F. Jackson

Nancy F. Jackson is a marriage and family therapist in private practice. In addition to her work with families and individuals, she conducts Social Effectiveness Training groups for children and consults with local school district personnel. She is coauthor of *Getting Along With Others: Teaching Social Effectiveness to Children* and has presented papers and workshops on social skills and children. She holds a master's degree and teaching credentials in special education and is a clinical member of the American Association for Marriage and Family Therapy.

Marcia L. Bennett

Marcia L. Bennett has a master's degree in psychology from Western Michigan University and a doctorate in psychology from the University of Nevada, Reno. She has worked in the field of developmental disabilities since 1973 and is currently Psychologist for Sierra Developmental Center in Reno. She is an instructor in workshops on Social Effectiveness Training and teaches social effectiveness to adolescent and adult clients living in community homes and at the developmental center.

Darden M. Bynum

Darden M. Bynum is Director of Community Services at Northern Nevada Mental Retardation Services. After earning a bachelor's degree from Vanderbilt University and a master's degree from the University of Alabama, he served for over 7 years as direct contact staff for people with disabilities. Currently, he is administering regional community programs. In addition to his role as a workshop presenter in Social Effectiveness Training, he conducts group training on the topics of social skills, personal relationships, and domestic violence.

Ellen Faryna

Ellen Faryna has worked in the field of developmental disabilities for 11 years. Her special interests include social skills training, sexuality education, and mental health services for clients and family members. She assisted in the introduction of Social Effectiveness Training to staff and clients in northern Nevada. Currently, she is working on her doctorate in clinical psychology at the California School of Professional Psychology in the San Francisco Bay Area.